To Lorrie —
Who is going
through a
storm of her
own —
with all good
wishes,
Barbara
Abercrombie

Also by Barbara Abercrombie

NOVELS
Good Riddance
Run for Your Life

BOOKS FOR YOUNG PEOPLE
The Other Side of a Poem
Amanda & Heather & Company
Cat-Man's Daughter
Charlie Anderson
Michael and the Cats
Bad Dog, Dodger!

Writing Out the Storm

Reading and Writing
Your Way Through
Serious Illness or Injury

BARBARA ABERCROMBIE

 ST. MARTIN'S GRIFFIN ⚓ NEW YORK

www.stmartins.com

Library of Congress, Cataloging-in-Publication Data
Abercrombie, Barbara.
   Writing out the storm : reading and writing your way through serious illness or injury / Barbara Abercrombie—1st ed.
      p.   cm.
   Includes bibliographical references (p. 107).
   ISBN 0-312-28545-0
   1. Creative writing—Therapeutic use.   2. Diaries—Therapeutic use.   3. Critically ill.   4. Terminally ill.   I. Title.

   RC489.W75 A24   2002
   615.8'515—dc21

                                                            200268367

First Edition: October 2002

10   9   8   7   6   5   4   3   2   1

*For R.V.A.,
husband, best friend,
with all my love*

Contents

Writing and reading decrease our sense of isolation. They deepen and widen and expand our sense of life: They feed the soul. When writers make us shake our heads with the exactness of their prose and their truths, and even make us laugh about ourselves or life, our buoyancy is restored. We are given a shot at dancing with, or at least clapping along with, the absurdity of life, instead of being squashed by it over and over again. It's like singing on a boat during a terrible storm at sea. You can't stop the raging storm, but singing can change the hearts and spirits of the people who are together on that ship.

—Anne Lamott, *Bird by Bird:*
Some Instructions on Writing and Life

INTRODUCTION

We read to know we are not alone.
—C. S. Lewis

The patient has to start by treating his illness not as a disaster, an occasion for depression or panic, but as a narrative, a story. Stories are antibodies against illness and pain.
—Anatole Broyard

The idea for this book began in a writing workshop I started four years ago at The Wellness Community in Los Angeles. People in the workshop ranged in age from early thirties to mid-eighties, and everyone, including me, had either recovered from cancer, was currently in treatment for it, or was a caregiver.

At the first session I began to expound on different genres of creative writing—how to transform experience and craft stories of having cancer into personal essays, fiction, or poems. I went on to the structure of a personal essay, the main elements of fiction, how to overcome the fear of writing. Everyone listened patiently and politely, but they all had the glazed look of people waiting for an overdue bus.

Finally, it dawned on me that I couldn't conduct the workshop the way I teach my regular creative writing classes. No one here cared about genre guidelines, no one needed or wanted pep talks for becoming a writer or advice on how to get published. They were here for writing as therapy, a way to deal emotionally with a life-threatening illness, a tool for finding a voice in a situation that leaves you feeling as if you have no control, no voice.

But how do you guide nonwriters into translating their feelings into words and going deeper into their own souls with language? You can't just say: Write about your fear of death, write about cancer, write about feeling desperate and crazy. You need a way in, you need to hear other voices telling their stories, you need guides and inspiration.

We finally found our guides, as well as inspiration, in poetry, memoir, and fiction. Writers like Raymond Carver, Alice Hoffman, Andre Dubus, Reynolds Price, to name just a few, who wrote about how they got through their illnesses and accidents, how it felt, what they discovered. Also nonwriters with high-profile stories of physical disaster and courage, like Christopher Reeve and Lance Armstrong. No simple slogans or platitudes, but deeply felt, eloquent renderings of emotions and situations we all knew to be true.

This book is an invitation for you to start writing, and it follows what we do in the workshop: Before each exercise I talk briefly about some aspect of my own experience with breast cancer, then we read aloud a poem or an excerpt from fiction or a memoir, and out of the reading, a word or a phrase or idea acts as a springboard for a five-minute writing exercise. After each exercise everyone reads their work aloud.

Why write? Because dealing with your emotions on paper can be a safe and private way to expose your feelings. Because the details of your life are precious and important and not to be lost. Because writing out painful emotions can also be good for your health.

In 1999 a study was reported in the *Journal of the American Medical Association* that linked writing to improved health for patients with asthma and rheumatoid arthritis. One group of patients wrote for twenty minutes over three consecutive days about the most stressful experience they ever had. A control group wrote about their plans for the day. When both groups were tested two weeks later, and then again at two and four months, those patients who were writing about painful events in their lives showed clinically relevant changes in their health compared to the control group. At the end of the article, the authors wrote: "This is the first study to demonstrate that writing about stressful life experiences improves physician ratings of disease severity and objective indices of disease severity in chronically ill patients."

The study was based on a method developed by psychologist James W. Pennebaker. In his book, *Opening Up*, Dr. Pennebaker reports testing the immune systems of two groups of students who wrote twenty minutes a day for four consecutive days. Like the study reported in the *Journal of the American Medical Association*, one group was told to write about superficial subjects, the other group to write about an extremely stressful event in their life. Blood samples from both groups were tested the day before writing, after the last writing session, then six weeks later. Dr. Pennebaker found that the students who wrote about painful, traumatic events showed heightened immune function and also paid fewer visits to the university's health center in the following weeks. "Writing helps to keep our psychological compass oriented," he says at the end of *Opening Up*. "Although not a panacea, writing can be an inexpensive, simple and sometimes painful way to help maintain our health."

In the workshop we soon realized that the written word read aloud also offered a deeper connection between people than simply talking.

In her essay, "The Literature of Personal Disaster," Nancy Mairs writes as she sits in her husband's hospital room about feeling trapped in "this profound and irrational solitude, as though walls of black glass had dropped on every side, shutting out the light . . ." And then asks, "Are we all groping for one another through our separate darks?"

Those of us who are ill or injured, or caring for someone who is, wrestle with our separate darks, our 3:00 A.M. terrors, the feeling of

insanity that comes from trying to live in a world of the healthy and
perfect while our own lives are overwhelmed with a physical ordeal.
We need all the comfort and solace, all the meaning and spirit we
can possibly find. Poetry, fiction, and autobiographical writing not
only can inspire us to write and offer new ways to express ourselves,
but also invites us into the company of people who have gone
through what we're going through. Writers who have mined their
own experiences for meaning and hope. Writers who can make us
laugh in recognition.

Our own writing is not only a release of emotion and a way to figure out what we think and feel, but it can also offer a path out of our
isolation; a way to reach through our own separate darks to give
words to what lies hidden in our souls.

Writing Out the Storm

SOMETHING HAPPENS

I'm in a waiting room surrounded by other women. A Muzak version of "People Will Say We're in Love" is playing. A woman in her late seventies sitting across from me with two friends is humming along with the music. A younger woman sitting next to me, wearing a scarf that covers her bald head, is writing Valentine cards. The walls of the waiting room are painted lavender. Sunlight spills through the open windows, and there's the smell of grass being mowed. It's oddly pleasant and peaceful here in this room filled with women of all ages, even though nobody's here for a good time.

The older woman's name is called, and when she's gone her two friends discuss her cooking. Apparently she's an excellent cook but doesn't have a grip on meatballs. Too dry, is the verdict. Somebody else they know puts two eggs in for one pound of meat. "It's gotta be soft like sausage soft," says one friend. "You have to work and work the meat. Put in seasonings. I only like Sylvia's meatballs."

I write all this down in a very small notebook. If I keep writing, I won't have to think about why I'm here.

My name is finally called. I'm here every year for an annual mammogram, I know the drill; no perfume or deodorant, sweater and bra off, jonny gown on and open in the front, my breast kneaded into position (those meatballs come to mind), then flattened rather alarmingly under a transparent vise. I hold my breath as the machine whirs.

Afterward I point out the lump next to my left nipple to the technician. I'm expecting a shrug, perhaps recognition of my hypochondria. Or even praise for being so alert, such a good girl for coming in right away to have it checked, even though this tiny lump that R. found yesterday is absolutely nothing. Instead the technician's face is serious as she feels the lump. Then she puts a little tag on it, kind of a breast Post-it, and schedules me for an immediate ultrasound exam.

I want to say: Look, I'm getting married in six months, I teach two courses and have a lot of students, I'm writing a novel. A major medical problem is not part of the plan. I really don't have time for this.

But of course I must have the ultrasound exam, and as I wait for it, sitting in another room still wearing the jonny gown top with the Post-it on my breast, I think how quickly life can swerve. Suddenly I'm being treated like a *patient*. I ran four miles this morning, I spent last weekend making love to my fiancé in Palm Springs, I'm teaching a three-hour class tonight. I'm not somebody who sits around in a damn jonny gown, a body part tagged, waiting for doctors. But I do wait, and I do have the exam. And then a doctor I've never met before tells me I need to see a breast surgeon right away to have the lump surgically removed and biopsied.

Something happens, and then the world spins on a new axis.

I am standing outside a shopping mall on a shimmering fall day in Chagrin Falls, Ohio, the name of the town portentous. I bend down to pick up my child, but the bending never finishes, breaks instead into spitting lights of pain that spread over a pool of half-consciousness. A tearing is felt—almost heard—within the thickness of flesh, moving in seconds across the base of the spine. The body instantly announces: This is an important event, this is an event you will never forget. I can't get up. The asphalt is icy. Somehow I am wedged into a car. The emergency room regrets not knowing what to do.

—Suzanne E. Berger, *Horizontal Woman*

Smith sees I'm awake and tells me help is on the way. He speaks calmly, even cheerily. His look, as he sits on his rock with his cane drawn across his lap, is one of pleasant commiseration: Ain't the two of us just had the shittiest luck? *it says. He and Bullet left the campground where they were staying, he later tells an investigator, because he wanted "some of those Marzes-bars they have up to the store." When I hear this little detail some weeks later, it occurs to me that I have nearly been killed by a character right out of one of my own novels. It's almost funny.*

—Stephen King, *On Writing, A Memoir of the Craft*

The doctors' faces were a professional grim. . . . *As they examined me the doctors exchanged, with their eyes, their verification of swollen lymph nodes in my neck. They talked their serious talk in the hall, and I could hear them when my children's chattering permitted me. I could hear the word* tumor.

I was full of plans for the future, like a tree of leaves. They fell off the branches at once, not blowing away, but laid at the root.

—Laurel Lee, *Walking Through the Fire, A Hospital Journal*

Whether you call it writing in a journal or keeping a notebook, buy yourself a beautiful book with blank pages, or buy a spiral notebook at the supermarket for $1.98. Or start a new file in your computer. There is no right or wrong way to do this. Just begin.

Start with the words *something happens*. See where they lead. Maybe you'll write about an accident or the start of an illness, the moment when your life spun on a new axis, when your plans began to fall like leaves. Or maybe you'll start with the description of a waiting room, the details of the moment, what you see and smell, hear and touch.

Ray Bradbury says the words he'd post in red letters ten feet high to encourage creativity are: WORK. RELAXATION. DON'T THINK.

If you keep your pen moving so fast you can't think, you'll begin to move out of your own way and connect to a deeper part of yourself.

You'll start writing about things you didn't even know that you knew or remembered. Trust the deep well of memory and knowledge and feeling you have. Write so fast, you won't hear that voice in your head carping that this is too boring to write about, too sentimental, too personal. The details of your life are valuable. Relax. Don't think. Keep writing.

THIS IS ONLY A TEST

The morning of the biopsy, R. and I have a long-standing appointment with the priest who's going to marry us. We discuss details of the service— our vows, the music, flowers, lighting the chapel with candles. We reserve the church for the evening of August 15, six months from now. I don't mention to the priest that we're going on to the hospital after this meeting, that I'm having a biopsy. It's like a very peculiar dream I'm having. Surgery in two hours. Even our wedding now seems to be an event we're only dreaming about.

Originally I'd thought of our eloping to Paris; I liked the sound of that. When I asked R. what he thought of this plan he said fine, but he wanted the kids to come, too. We have five children between us, all grown, all of whom have spouses or partners. Taking ten extra people to Paris seemed a little pricey to me and no longer terribly romantic.

When we became engaged last November, I grew nervous about our happiness. Were we too happy, too lucky? We both had work that we loved, healthy children, our own houses and enough money, and we were not only in love with each other but best friends; we'd known each other for twenty-eight years. I worried about paying off the gods; things were on such a roll for us that the gods might get jealous. R. said we had already paid them off—our first marriages falling apart and painful divorces, my mother's long illness and her death a year ago.

Then a few weeks later I lost the emerald out of my engagement ring. When I looked down at my hand and saw the empty space, it was like looking in the mirror and discovering a tooth missing.

Though I searched everywhere, I couldn't find it and finally, with mixed feelings, I told R. that the gods had been paid off.

Now on this warm, sunny February morning, we stop in the chapel before driving to the hospital. I've come here for eight o'clock Communion on Sundays off and on through the years, and last year we had a small family memorial service in the chapel for my mother. I don't think of myself as religious, but I love the Episcopal Church, the ritual, the language, the music, and I love this small stone chapel. I believe that there is something here, something beyond the material world, a spiritual mystery I can't figure out.

I have this strange sense of fate—if I have cancer, I have it, and prayers not to have it seem a little late. Is this lack of faith, or simply being realistic? Twenty-five years ago I was with my mother-in-law, who was the same age as I am now, when she died of cancer. Though I still come to church on occasion, I lost the comfort of an easy faith when she died, the belief that all would turn out for the best if you prayed hard enough. On my knees now in a pew, I pray for the only thing that seems reasonable: courage.

But surely the gods can't be this jealous, life can't be this ironic. *After all these years she finally gets her act together and then boom—the big C.* No, this is just a biopsy I'm having, this is just a test.

You notice the swell of one of your breasts, and notice it again weeks later. When you direct his hand to it, his eyebrows slant into worry. He says, "You even swell swell," but he is the one who insists you call your gynecologist in the morning.

She sends you to a surgeon, who doesn't like what he feels. A few mornings later, the surgeon does the biopsy. The pathology lab will have your results in a week.

Meanwhile, your boyfriend reads Dr. Love's book and reports that the odds of getting cancer at your age are almost one in three thousand. He says, "You're not the one."

You keep telling yourself, "This is only a test," but that week of waiting for the results is an unrelieved high-pitched tone. Then you are told that it is a real emergency.

Too late, you realize that your body was perfect—every healthy body is.

—Melissa Bank, *The Girls' Guide to Hunting and Fishing*

. . . a small lump no one is worried about is biopsied, just to see. There are precancerous changes in the cells and we move the activity up a notch. I enter a time of winter darkness, taxis whisking me and my slides around New York into the Persian-rug-spread waiting rooms of Park Avenue brownstones and up and down the glass and marble corridors of Memorial Sloan-Kettering Hospital. The doctors agree: why not? It becomes obvious that they have no real answers for this: they cannot cure, they can merely catch it in time. A week before the surgery, I suddenly panic. I cannot do this. I am too young, I am wearing blue jeans, I have a Bloomingdale's charge card.

—Annette Williams Jaffee, "The Good Mother" from *Living on the Margins, Women Writers on Breast Cancer*

In Ethiopia, illness is an opportunity. It is something to contemplate. It invites the sick person to undertake an internal spiritual and healing journey. It provides a possibility for growth. The sick person is a seeker, a voyager, an explorer. And the word can cure. Illness can be experienced, expressed, and understood, but only in the way that one understands a mystery, for that, in part, is what illness is.

—Louise DeSalvo, *Writing As a Way of Healing*

Write the words: *this is only a test . . .* and follow wherever they go. If you veer off into another topic, that's fine, just keep going.

Write about being too young for this.

In the workshop Laura writes: *I'm definitely too young to have cancer— diagnosed at 44! Scared the shit out of my peers and friends who were younger . . . I am too young to have cancer . . . Yet when I am old, I will look back to the distant memory of the cancer I had. The year of shallow breathing and tightened throat.*

Laura's husband Bob writes: *This period is only a test. I'm too young, too unprepared, too busy for this stage of life. I want it over. Now! I've learned plenty. I'm sure I'm a better person for this episode already . . . dealing with cancer has been a pervasive part of the past year . . . My intention was to back off on other pursuits, but it doesn't happen. The Patient herself sets the worst example. Care for the kids needs to be better than before to avoid the nagging fear of them having suffered. The meals, the schedule must be more perfect. There is no emotional energy left to handle it and make up for small disappointments. Also the persistent fear that this month may be the last with some version of reasonable health. If it's just a test, it's going on far too long. Somebody wake up the proctor!*

Forget what you were taught in English class. You have permission to throw out all the grammar you ever learned and to make up your own spelling. Someday, if you ever think about getting published, then you can let the carping editor in your head loose on the page to make sense of your grammar and give structure to what you write. But that's the second step. And you can't get there without the first step.

A student once told me that little girls in Russia who want to join the ballet are not allowed to study technique until they're nine years old. Up until then they're encouraged to dance on their own, to have fun and feel free.

This is a wonderful analogy for writing. Don't think about technique right now. Dance. Sing. Fool around on the page.

Elizabeth writes: *Writing helps me share the music of my life.*

What would the sound track for your life be? Garth Brooks, a Puccini aria, heavy metal, Dave Matthews, a Mozart sonata? Write about the music of your own life.

3

WHAT THE DOCTOR SAID

*V*alentine's Day 1997. *I've always thought this was one of those hyped holi-*days, meant to sell a lot of candy and flowers, like Mother's Day, that causes vast numbers of people who don't have a lover, or a mother or a child, to feel depressed and left out. Consumerism at its emotional worst. In spite of my bad attitude about Valentine's Day, R. has given me a present—a beautiful watch; I can hear it ticking on my wrist.

It's an overcast afternoon, the good weather of yesterday has turned gray and damp and chilly. If you were writing this scene as fiction you wouldn't put in that detail; it's too obvious, a cliché.

Newsweek has a big cover story this week on breast cancer, and I read it as we wait in the kitchen for my surgeon to call with the results of the biopsy. He was quite sure that it wasn't cancer and that we'd have the results right away. But it's been twenty-four hours now.

My left breast, the breast that was biopsied yesterday, now wearing a Band-Aid, doesn't hurt so much as feel heavy and dangerous. Somewhere in a lab there's this tiny piece of me on a slide being examined under a microscope by strangers, and what they find will determine my future. Whether, in fact, I have a future.

My new watch ticks in the silence. If this were fiction, I'd make a big deal out of the ticking; I'd turn it into a metaphor. Though of course this, too, would be a pretty obvious cliché. The pages of *Newsweek* rustle as I turn them. R. does paperwork next to me at the kitchen table.

Finally, the phone rings.

So sorry but it's bad news, says the doctor, it's cancer and he was so sure I didn't have cancer but it is cancer and he's so sorry. His voice goes on and on as the kitchen tilts. R. holds me. I cry. I feel like I'm in a very bad movie.

He said it doesn't look good
he said it looks bad in fact real bad
he said I counted thirty-two of them on one lung before
I quit counting them
I said I'm glad I wouldn't want to know
about any more being there than that
he said are you a religious man do you kneel down
in forest groves and let yourself ask for help
when you come to a waterfall
mist blowing against your face and arms
do you stop and ask for understanding at those moments
I said not yet but I intend to start today
He said I'm real sorry he said
I wish I had some other kind of news to give you
I said Amen and he said something else
I didn't catch and not knowing what else to do
and not wanting him to have to repeat it
and me to have to fully digest it
I just looked at him
for a minute and he looked back it was then
I jumped up and shook hands with this man who'd just given me
something no one else on earth had ever given me
I may even have thanked him habit being so strong
        —Raymond Carver, "What the Doctor Said,"
            from *A New Path to the Waterfall*

When the doctors came in—a pair of them, the intern and the pulmonary man—they stayed as close to each other as they could, like puppies. They stood at his bedside, for the new enlightenment demands that a doctor not deliver doom from the foot of the bed, looming like God. The intern spoke: "Mr. Horwitz, we have the results of the bronchoscopy. It does show evidence of pneumocystis in the lungs."

Was there a pause for the world to stop? There must have been, because I remember the crack of silence. Roger staring at the two men. Then he simply shut his eyes, and only I, who was the rest of him, could see how stricken was the stillness in his face.

—Paul Monette, *Borrowed Time, An AIDS Memoir*

So much of a writer's life consists of assumed suffering, rhetorical suffering, that I felt something like relief, even elation, when the doctor told me that I had cancer of the prostate. Suddenly there was in the air a rich sense of crisis—real crisis, yet one that also contained echoes of ideas like the crisis of language, the crisis of literature, or of personality. It seemed to me that my existence, whatever I thought, or did, had taken on a kind of meter, as in poetry or in taxis.

—Anatole Broyard, *Intoxicated by My Illness*

I was certain my doctor was phoning me to tell me the biopsy had come back negative, I was absolutely sure of it, but then she said, "Alice, I'm so sorry." I could hear the concern and sadness in her voice, and I understood that some things are true no matter how and when you're told. In a single moment the world as I knew it dropped away from me, leaving me on a far and distant planet, one where there was no gravity and no oxygen and nothing made sense anymore.

—Alice Hoffman, "Sustained by Fiction
While Facing Life's Facts," *New York Times*

Write about what the doctor said to you. Did he or she loom over you like God and quote statistics or act like a human being? Or was the doctor just a voice over the telephone? What were your first thoughts? What could you see out the window? What time of year was it? Write about the world stopping. Write about suddenly being on a far and distant planet.

In the workshop Nancy writes: *The doctor said, "I've seen some cases live fifteen to twenty years." Excuse me? Excuse me? Some cases? What the fuck is that? Some cases?*

Neva writes: *I was lying on a gurney in the hospital, I was sedated so it was in many ways like a bad dream. The doctor leaned over the railing and said, You have cancer . . . It was as though my body was on fire and bleeding. I was scared and very afraid of dying. Of course, I knew I was going to die. All the literature and propaganda we hear as non-cancer patients links death as the direct result of cancer. The only question I had was when. There was no "if" I die.*

When you write down details of a bad time, you connect to the moment, you're taking notes, you have to pay attention to what's going on. You write down the words the doctor says, the details of the room you're in, the clothes you're wearing, and the thoughts racing through your head. You stay focused. And at the same time you're also the observer recording this. Writing can give you a sense of distance and control.

Dave writes about what the doctor said in a scene he imagines took place right after his surgery: *. . . walking down the hall, first words to a waiting wife who is leaning forward, eyes wide open, ears wanting not to close, mouth caulked shut—"Your husband is obese, he made it too hard." Seeing the wife's caulked shut mouth and seeking eyes, he added, "He will be in recovery for awhile. He is down the hall. Labs aren't back yet but only one lymph node looked bad, better than we expected."*

Later he writes: *The metallic taste wouldn't leave my mouth, as the C word hung cauterized, ragged edge by ragged edge . . . My tears began, flowing over my unshaven face. For who could shave day after day?*

In the workshop we start each session with a list of bad moments since the last meeting, then a list of pleasures.

Make a list of the painful moments of the past week. Maybe an examination, or someone being insensitive or making too many demands on you, or problems at work or at home. After you make the list, choose one item on it and write about it for five minutes.

Now make a list of pleasures from the past week. A card from a friend, a cup of coffee, a sunset, a kiss—whatever moments gave you pleasure this week. Again, choose one thing from the list and write about it for five minutes.

Making a list can be a way to get into your writing when you don't have a lot of energy. It can also be a way to ease into difficult territory.

Laura lists what the doctor said:

You can't have another lump in your neck, it's only scar tissue from the incision.

You neck can drain, just keep it clean.

I don't have the final test results.

I called the pathologist. He says It looks like lymphoma.

Sometimes from the images and memories that surface in quick five-minute writing exercises, deeper writing evolves.

Nancy, who is married to a doctor, later writes a poem entitled "Diagnosed."

> *Monday at the hospital,*
> *waiting in the exam room my chart reads, r/o lymphoma.*
> *The words seem to grow before my eyes.*
> *The earth stops revolving,*
> *I can't breathe,*
> *the doctor finds more nodes.*

It can't be true. I'm very healthy.
I take my vitamins and watch my diet, most of the time.
I even exercise, when I think about it.
I'll get the biopsy—they'll all be wrong.
Besides, I'm a nurse, not a patient.

Deny. Off to surgery.

Deny. Home waiting days for the results.
I'll see the doctor in the morning.

But when Glenn comes home he is wearing sadness.
The earth stops once again as our eyes meet.

"I have it don't I?"

"Yes, my darling, I'm afraid you do."

4

TIME IS A MOUNTAIN LION

R. comes with me to see the surgeon who did the biopsy. I've been studying *Dr. Susan Love's Breast Book*, and I'm armed with a long list of questions and a tape recorder. I like this doctor; his energy cranks mine up another notch. He spends a lot of time talking to us, he's not threatened by my tape recorder and notebook, and he has his kids' artwork framed and hung on his office walls.

He recommends that I have a lumpectomy instead of a mastectomy, followed by radiation. When he does the lumpectomy he'll check the margins of the tumor and do a lymph node dissection to see if the cancer has spread. The results of this surgery, including more tests on the tumor that was removed during the biopsy, will tell us if it's an aggressive form of breast cancer and if I need chemotherapy.

Afterward, when we're going down in the elevator, two women get on with a cart piled with pamphlets. "Hi," says one brightly, holding a pamphlet out to us. "You want to read about Hospice?" I'm scared I'm going to die, and here are these helpful ladies with information on how to get through it. To their consternation, as well as R.'s, I start to laugh; though maybe the sound is closer to hysteria than laughter.

On the way home in the car I say to R., "You don't have to marry me if I don't have any eyebrows."

He pats my hand. "I'm not marrying you for your eyebrows."

"If I have to have chemo, I'll be bald for the wedding." I have this nightmare vision of myself looking like an egg at the altar.

"You can wear a wig," he says.

But even if I have to have chemo, I know I'm lucky because the tumor is small. Thanks to R. it was found early. Joanna, my sister-in-law, was just diagnosed with breast cancer a few weeks ago, so I checked myself (I was months overdue for a mammogram and lazy about examining myself every month) but I didn't find anything. I asked R. to check.

"Here's something," he said. It was the size of a pea, next to my left nipple.

"Well, it takes an engineer to find these things," I said. He didn't think I was funny.

"Get a mammogram," he said, and I said yes, even though I was sure it was nothing. Oddly, the lump never did show up on that mammogram I just had.

I called Joanna earlier this morning. "You're not going to believe this," I said.

In the middle of the night when I can't sleep I write in my journal. Nothing very articulate, just fear and attempts at bravado. I haven't written in my journal all week because I didn't want to add those words *I have a lump in my breast to* my history. I don't want to write the C word in my journal. Instead I've been writing notes down on tiny scraps of paper, like I'm whispering, like none of this is valid or quite real.

I have over fifty of these spiral, college-lined notebooks that I call my journal. Who will read them if I die? Would R. want to? Do I want my daughters to read them? Do I have time to rewrite all of them so I'll appear to be a better person, less neurotic, more coura-geous and generous? I'm too old to die young, I may just die *early*.

At 3:00 A.M. I wake R. up to tell him that I'm afraid I'm going to die. "You can't die," he says, half-sleep, "You're getting married next summer." I don't buy his logic, but I love his calm conviction, his constant sweetness and goodness toward me, even when I wake him at 3:00 A.M. I know how some men can't handle illness and fear, and as a consequence they turn cold and distant. But R. has become more loving if anything.

I try to crowd out my fear by writing a list in my journal of blessings and pleasures. Every morning this week R. and I have made love, able to turn off the fear, and exist simply in our bodies, not in our minds. This is at the top of my list.

My initial experience of illness was as a series of disconnected shocks, and my first instinct was to try to bring it under control by turning it into a narrative. Always in emergencies we invent narratives. . . . Storytelling seems to be a natural reaction to illness. . . . Metaphor was one of my symptoms. I saw my illness as a visit to a disturbed country, rather like contemporary China. I imagined it as a love affair with a demented woman who demanded things I had never done before.
       —Anatole Broyard, *Intoxicated by My Illness*

When samurai warriors went into battle, they carried a little purse containing the money for their funeral and everything that was necessary. If you go into a battle fearlessly accepting the possibility of death and almost embracing it, you have a much better chance of fighting well, and in fact of winning, than if you go into battle scared of death. I think a lot of Buddhist and spiritual practice in general is aimed at removing the fear of our own death. The fear of our own death is like the fear of our own birth or the fear of our own life.
  —Rick Fields, "I Live a Disease Threatening Life," from *Inner Fire*

In the middle of the night, with moonlight streaming in and Margaret beside me, it seemed hard to believe that something inside me was trying its damnedest to kill me. I shut my eyes and tried to sleep again. I felt as if there were a stranger in the bed with us. The stranger, of course, was cancer.
     —Michael Korda, *Man to Man, Surviving Prostate Cancer*

There's a game called Smoke in which one player thinks of a famous person and all the other players ask questions to discover the identity of this person. The questions have to be framed in metaphor: If this person were smoke, what kind would he or she be? If this person were an eating utensil, a piece of music, weather, animal, jewelry, a car? The famous person is more often guessed than not.

Metaphor is about connectedness; it is simply comparing two very different things to point up the connection.

In a poem called "Woman Bathing," Raymond Carver, who was ill at the time, writes of a joyful day spent in sunlight with the woman he loves, laughing at nothing, and asks the rhetorical question of how long do they have left together. Later there's a line, a metaphor, that makes this question come alive: *Time is a mountain lion.*

Well, we all know on one level that makes no sense, at least not logical sense; time is one thing and mountain lions a whole other subject. But this line gives me the *feeling* that time is after me, coming down the mountain fast, and there's no stopping it. It's dangerous and powerful and headed right at me. *Time is a mountain lion* might mean something totally different to you; there's no one way, no right way, to interpret it.

We know that illness is far different than a love affair with a demented partner demanding things we've never done before, as Anatole Broyard compares it to. But it goes deeper, we understand it on an emotional level. And *emotionally* it makes sense if you've ever gone through procedures demanded in a hospital, wanting to please, yet your body recoiling at every request.

Try writing some metaphors. Metaphor can be a way to go deeper into your own feelings because you don't feel as exposed.

Imagine fear as an animal. Whatever your mind flashes on. There's no correct answer, it's not a test. This is your fear, no one else's.

When you touch this animal, what does it feel like? Smell like? What does it eat? What does it need in order to thrive? What can tame it?

Beatrice writes that her fear is a snake . . . *his slippery mass has noise-lessly coiled around my heart like a tourniquet. He gobbles down my opti-*

mism, gorges on my dreams, devours my self-esteem and sinks his fangs into my core, poisoning me with self-doubt, anxiety, feelings of failure and doom.

Laura's fear is a parasite—so small she cannot be seen with the naked eye. She crawls through my stomach and gut and up into my throat and squeezes me with constricting pain . . . My pain and fear give pleasure to the fear parasite. She can even cross the blood-brain barrier and get into my brain. My fear parasite clouds my vision and brings darkness. My fear parasite bathes in my tears.

Write about hope. If hope were music, what kind would it be? What if hope were a pair of shoes, a car, a sound or a smell, a meal? Sarah writes, *Hope is like breakfast. It gets you through the day.*

What does the word *healing* making you think of? If it were something else, what would it be?

Margie writes, *If healing were music, it would be the chimes from the nearby Catholic church ringing the hour . . . constant . . . steady . . . dependable.*

5

ATTENDING YOUR OWN
MEMORIAL SERVICE

You're sure I'm not bothering you?" asks Susan when she calls to see how I am.

I tell her of course not; I love hearing from her. My long friendship with Susan and another colleague, Sunny, doesn't depend on constant connection. We might not talk for months when we're all busy writing and teaching, but we can always pick up wherever we leave off. I called them both in the beginning, asking them to be on standby to cover my classes if I couldn't teach. Now Sunny and Susan call regularly.

I love hearing from all my friends and family. Talking to everybody boosts my mood, makes me do my brave cancer patient act. When I make jokes and tell them how fine I feel, I actually begin to feel that way.

Of course this doesn't happen, everybody calling and helping you to feel good, unless you let everybody know what's going on. I told people close to me about it in stages:

"I've got this little lump . . ." (Along with my "it takes an engineer" line.)

"It's just a biopsy." (And then how my doctor is almost *positive* it's not malignant.)

"It's just a very tiny little tumor and was found really, really early." (I talk really, really fast at this stage because people are always so horrified hearing the word *cancer*, instantly equating it with death.)

My daughters and sons-in-law, my about-to-be brother and sister-in-law, my former in-laws, my future stepchildren, my brother, my cousins, my close friends—they all visit or keep calling to check on me, or they send notes or e-mail messages. I even get a phone call from my ex-husband, who is in Turkey, and a note from R's ex-wife in New Hampshire.

It's like being around for your own memorial service.

Of course some people don't call or write, don't know what to say or do. Or stumble into a cancer disaster story as they're talking to you, or tell you a lot of New Age stuff about your wounded inner child that you really don't want to hear about right now. Or are afraid of disturbing you. Or simply can't be around cancer for whatever reason. But when your body is in serious trouble, you realize life is just too short to worry about who does or doesn't call. Those who do, you cherish and spend your energy on. You cut your losses, whatever they may be, and move on.

It was extraordinary, the outpouring of sympathy and concern, how people would call, then call again, especially considering the difficulty of a situation that changed from hour to hour, and to which I could give no name. Cancer and a stroke we can at least pretend are known quantities: there are hundreds of success stories, miracles of therapy, remission, cure. But confronted with this ever-changing misery, there were no words. Yet they found them, my friends, mysteriously, abundantly . . .

There are people you hardly know who suddenly surface, a sort of underground of "resistance workers" who are geniuses at this sort of thing, and others whom you do know but who unexpectedly blossom as caregivers.

—Molly Haskell, *Love and Other Infectious Diseases*

Each post brought new letters: letters of sympathy, letters of encouragement, letters from people I hadn't spoke to, or heard from, in years. And when I wasn't bombarded by the past, I found I was alone with a rather interesting person, someone I had never spent much time alone with: myself.

—Robert McCrum, *My Year Off, Recovering Life After a Stroke*

. . . I started dialing wildly—my sister, my dad, my college roommate, my next door neighbor, my dear friend Lori. Not one single person was home. I had just heard that I had cancer and everyone was at the grocery store or at the gym or on the road home from work. Why weren't they instantly and totally available to hear my news? I blurted the fact of my cancer on message machines all across the country. It was more important for me to tell than to engage in any kind of a dialogue. I wanted the news out of me, where it felt like it would do less harm.

—Jennie Nash, *The Victoria's Secret Catalog Never Stops Coming*

What do you need from your friends and family? Write a letter to someone you love saying all the things you can't say in real life, all the hard things that need to be said. Remember: You don't have to mail it.

Ligaya comes to Los Angeles from the Philippines to be with her mother, who has stomach cancer. Her mother didn't want to join the workshop, but Ligaya comes to each meeting to write about her own frustrations, anger, and fears. She writes her mother a long letter, pouring out reflections about her childhood, questions about herself, *Why do I get angry easily? Why am I so critical to people? Why am I not a loving person? Why is it very hard for me to smile, to laugh?* and fears about her mother's health, *The treatment that you're getting now will not have its full effect on you if you will not be able to manage your negative emotions . . . I'm here to support you but if you will not do anything to release all your anger in your life, then our efforts will just be wasted . . . You have a right to be happy and enjoy life. You have gone through a lot of crisis in your life and you have survived them all . . .* She ends the letter with admonitions to her mother to treat her grandchildren differently, *May you be gentle and loving with them, avoid harassing them; avoid being angry with them. May you learn to express your love to them, learn to really communicate with them and build a closer, loving relationship with them.*

At the next workshop meeting Ligaya tells us she gave the letter to her mother. There's an audible gasp from the group. "She got so angry," Ligaya says, "she felt I was too ungrateful for all the sacrifices she made for the family. She was crying, and isolated herself in her room for three days."

And then they talked. Ligaya tells us: ". . . she said she was not aware that she was not nurturing us . . . she was concerned with there always being enough food on the table, money to give us for our snacks at school and all the daily needs at home . . . She didn't know what mothering really entails; poverty really isolated her and limited her in all aspects of life."

Months later Ligaya e-mails me from the Philippines: "Mama told me she writes now how she feels and what she thinks. So little by little, she's getting out of herself and is now trying to express herself."

Laura writes a letter to someone newly diagnosed, in which she shares her own cancer story, lists books that helped her, information about The Wellness Community, then ends the letter with this paragraph:

Another thing I did at the time of my diagnosis was to contact more than 75 of my friends and acquaintances to let them know. It will take everyone time to process what you have told them, but they will be in a better position to help you if they know. I think it was easier for my friends to hear from me because I can sound cheerful and amusing even when I don't feel that way. I have been overwhelmed by so many friends helping me with prayers, cards, gifts, flowers, visits, phone calls, emotional support, meals, laundry, free massages, driving me and my children, etc. etc. When things are tough, I remember all the kind gestures and the people who love me.

Write about how you tell people about what you're going through— or how you keep it secret.

Write about people's reactions when you tell them the truth.

Write about the consequences of reaching out—or not reaching out.

Valerie writes: *When I was young the word cancer was whispered, but I tell everyone. Who knows what helpful things you might find out. And so often the response is, "Oh, my mother (daughter, husband, cousin, etc.) had or has cancer too." Some people of course don't know what to say, but that's okay. I heard about a woman who was treated for breast cancer for seven years and never let her husband know. How on earth did she do that? What a missed opportunity for comfort for her and for him to show his caring. My husband has sat through every test, doctor's appointment and every chemotherapy session. My family and friends have shown their support in countless ways. How sad if I and they had missed that. We not only care for those we love, we learn to love even more those we care for.*

6

A Bull Pen of Patients

A lumpectomy is an outpatient procedure, and as things go at a hospital, not a big deal. For the patients who are waiting for day surgery, after being called in from the main waiting room, there's kind of a bull pen. A row of beds lined up against the wall for those about to go into the operating room, and then some chairs for patients who are scheduled later. This group of later patients, of which I am now a member, are to sit in Naugahyde chairs opposite the beds in this large, noisy, busy room wearing just a jonny gown and underwear, clutching our belongings in a plastic bag.

A nurse hands me the gown and tells me to get undressed in the ladies' room. "When will a bed be free?" I ask.

"In about an hour."

"Okay, I'll get undressed then."

"You have to do it now."

"Why?"

"Because these are the rules."

"I'm not getting undressed until a bed is ready," I say.

Other nurses are called in—a whole Greek chorus of them telling me *these are the rules.* I know these are the rules because when I had the biopsy last week I sat out here feeling like I was in one of those nightmares in which you've forgotten your clothes and you're in public trying to act as if everything is cool. There's no dignity. It's like bad police procedure, when they strip search someone so the person will know who's in charge.

So now I simply refuse to go along with their rules, I refuse to sit in a public place wearing just my undies and a jonny gown. I may have these cells going out of control in my body, but I can at least be in charge of this situation. "Let me know when a bed is ready," I say, sitting in a Naugahyde chair with all my clothes on. The nurses give me dirty looks, but what can they do, rip my clothes off?

I think of my mother in the hospital last year. There was nothing more the doctors could do for her except keep her comfortable, so the hospital wanted to move her out of critical care to another floor, where she'd have to have a roommate. "Under no circumstances am I going to share a room," said my mother, eighty-seven years old and weighing ninety-five pounds.

"But these are the rules," said her doctors, one after another, each trying to convince her to move. "You can't have this room any longer."

"Well, then, I'm going home," she said. And she did.

The anesthesiologist is very enthusiastic about his job, more like a choreographer or a film director than a doctor. "Tell me what you want, and I'll tell you what I have," he says.

This isn't so bad; my very own designer drug dealer. I tell him I want to feel relaxed with no pain, I don't want to feel anxious, and I don't want to be sick afterward.

"Knock and block!" he says.

"I ran four miles this morning," I tell him. I don't want him to think I'm someone who lies around on a gurney, pleading for oblivion.

After the lumpectomy, high and happy on the drugs, with tubes hanging from my armpit into a drain bottle, which, when I put my jacket over it, juts out looking like I had a weird boob job that missed the mark, we go home.

Like so many health services offered to the poor, this clinic's emphasis seemed more on punishment through waiting than relief by cure. The building was a pretty Beaux Arts schoolhouse, tucked among mature

*sycamores at Chelsea's edge. It was now reduced from primary
education to basic regret. Barred and wired like a zoo, it was.*

*The waiting room accosted us losers with overbright posters. I felt
sufficiently ashamed without DOES IT BURN WHEN YOU MAKE
WATER? IF SO, YOU PROBABLY HAVE . . . a long list of fine print
followed, spikey Latin names for what now crimped our love lives.*

—Allan Gurganus, *Plays Well with Others*

*Becoming completely dependent on other people is a terrible adjustment
to make. I lay there for a month floating among various moods and
feelings—gratitude, horror, self-pity, confusion, anger. There was one
doctor at UVA who was the bane of my existence. She came in at all
hours of the day and night to poke and prod . . . She would also talk to
me as if I were three. Finally, I couldn't stand it anymore. I yelled, "Fuck
you, I'm a forty-two-year-old man. You treat me like one or don't come
in this room again." That chastened her a little bit. I know she intended
no harm or discomfort, but she increased my feelings of despair and
loss, humiliation and embarrassment.*

—Christopher Reeve, *Still Me*

*You reach for the pitcher or cup and do not touch it. You roll toward
the table and extend your arm; if you are in traction you cannot truly
roll; you just turn a bit. You still cannot touch the plastic pitcher or
paper cup. With one hand you hold the table and pull it toward you,
then turn it this way or that until its angle brings your drink closer.
Finally you can touch the side of the vessel, carefully turn it in a series
of partial circles until it is within range. Then you hold it and pour
from it or bring it to your lips. This is also true of the small paper
container that holds your pills. The nurses place them, too, just out
of reach. Not every time, but enough of the time, enough. Hospital
challenge.*

—Andre Dubus, "Sketches at Home," from *Broken Vessels.*

*When she emerged, in a hospital gown, the sight shocked me. She had
been shapely and sexy in her skirt and sweater; now, in the loose gown,*

she was without form. I had never thought until that moment how
utterly and completely people give up their individuality and control
when they become patients. They're told, "Sit here. Fill out these forms.
Stick out your arm. Lie down. Open your mouth." They enter a world
with a strange language and unfamiliar rules, in which they are no
longer in control. They don't even have their clothes to provide identity. I
saw that it was certainly humbling, probably frightening, and perhaps
humiliating to be so totally under the command of others. My reaction
spoke volumes about what patients sacrifice in dignity and self-esteem,
and what I, as a doctor, had not seen quite this way before.

—Sidney J. Winawer, M.D., *Healing Lessons*

Nancy comes to a workshop session one day and announces that
she's broken the rule about not letting anyone read your journal or
notebook. I suggested this rule of guarding the privacy of your notebook because we're so vulnerable when we write—all our thoughts
and feelings and fantasies and experiences are right out there, naked
with no place to hide. Anne Lamott calls writing ". . . a pretty desperate endeavor, because it's about some of our deepest needs: our
need to be visible, to be heard, our need to make sense of our lives,
to wake up and grow and belong."

Nancy tells us she gave her whole journal to her daughter to read.
"It was the only way I could tell her what I'm going through," she says.

I had never considered before that your most private writing
could be a necessary bridge to those closest to you, especially when
you're in pain or trouble. Nancy taught us all a valuable lesson.

Though not everyone's experience is the same. Gloria pours out
such raw anger and pain on the page that she's terrified of the possibility of her family ever reading what she's writing. Her solution is to
tear out pages of her journal and burn them. She says the act of writing is the important thing for her, not making a record of what she's
going through.

Think about whether you'll invite the people closest to you to read your notebook, or show them something you've written. Or will you burn every word? Or maybe something in between? Make up your own rules about this.

Deb writes a poem:

> *Show me something you have written,*
> *a piece of life*
> *you have bitten*
> *off*
> *to make your book*
> *of love and loss.*
>
> *Open drawers to*
> *pages hidden,*
> *show me something you have written.*

Write about feeling vulnerable. Write about following the rules. Write about not following the rules.

Write about taking control.

Ginny writes: *It's 6:30 am. I am surrounded by white coats and heads and I hear, "This is Mrs. S., neck dissection." At that moment my thinking and mind cleared from all the drugs and pain. "I am not a neck dissection. My name is Ginny." The next morning, as the wizards of Westwood gathered around me, I wrote down, "My name is Ginny and what I need to hear is some hope and good news. Remember who I am."*

Write the words: *Remember who I am . . .* and follow where they lead.

7

HELD AT GUNPOINT

*M*y *friends are praying for me: Jews, Episcopalians, Mormons, Buddhists,*
Catholics, born-agains, even the atheists say they're praying.

My prayers are more to the point now: Don't let me die.

Do I have faith that these prayers are being heard? And if so, by
whom? The word *faith* suddenly sounds fuzzy, a bit out of focus.
Like I'm floating prayers heavenward on little puffs of clouds when I
pray. I do believe in the meditation aspect of prayer and the notion of
positive energy from prayer flowing out into the universe. I believe
in miracles, too. I'm just not sure of the cause and effect angle.

At night I have strange dreams: I'm flying high up in the sky in a
very small dangerous contraption with no room to maneuver. In
another dream I'm held at gunpoint. Then I appear at a party
attended by my ex-husband wearing only my bathrobe. My friend
Ruth, who's a psychotherapist, once told me I have the most obvious
dreams of anyone she knows.

There are moments when I walk wordlessly up to R., fold myself
into his arms, and weep.

Good weather again, sunny and warm as summer. We sit on the
deck at his house in Palos Verdes; he reads, and I write in my journal. The ocean shines blue in the distance, his early-spring garden
blooms all around us. A few years ago, R. sent me a poem by Rumi
that began with the words: *Come to the garden in the spring . . .*

We're once again waiting for the phone to ring with news, waiting to hear the results of the lymph node dissection and tissue
examination. Are cancer cells, like tiny terrorists, loose and racing

through my body at this very moment? I take deep yoga breaths. Test results hold you hostage as you wait for the phone to ring.

I write in my journal that if the cancer has spread, and I need chemo, I'll buy Tina Turner wigs and some very cool new outfits. And I'll sit out here on the deck every afternoon and smoke pot.

My future stepson stops by and gives me a bouquet of wildflowers he's picked, and my heart is touched.

There's a moment midafternoon when I feel such absolute peace; all will be fine. And then later, nothing but fear. I've never felt pure terror before. It *is* like being held at gunpoint.

When the call comes that everything is okay so far, negative nodes and nothing in the margin tissue, I feel a blast of joy, gratitude, and relief. "You still might need chemo," says my surgeon. "You won't know for sure until you see the oncologist, but so far things are looking good."

We go out to dinner to celebrate my negative nodes and clean margins. A week ago I didn't even know what nodes and margins were.

There's a full moon, and I love every house that's shining in the moonlight, every blade of grass, rock, tree, flower, animal. I remember Emily's lines from *Our Town* after she returns from the dead to say good-bye to the things she'd taken for granted, about how sweet and good life is but the living never realize this.

Tonight I take nothing for granted. I realize how sweet and good life is, how fragile the celebrations.

... *the numbers were all-important for me, and I would wait nervously by the phone for every result. I picked up right away.*

"We got the blood counts back," LaTrice said.

"Yeah?" I said nervously.

"Lance, they're normal," she said.

I held the thought up in my mind and looked at it: I was no longer sick. I might not stay that way; I still had a long year ahead of me, and

if the illness returned it would probably happen in the next 12 months.
But for this moment, at least for this brief and priceless moment, there
wasn't a physical trace of cancer left in my body.

—Lance Armstrong, *It's Not About the Bike*

After a heart attack, you feel as if someone has broken into the
house in the middle of the night. You know there is a killer waiting
in the dark basement. You imagine him mounting the stairs with
a knife in his hands. You finger the tiny glass cylinder of nitro as
if it were Kryptonite. You rub the middle of your chest and feel
the bumpy scars where the bone was wired back together after bypass.

—Lance Morrow, "Lessons of a Bad Heart," *Time* 3/19/01

If you are flung over a horse's head, you very well might break your
neck. It just happens. But where God comes in, where grace enters, is in
the strength you find to deal with it. You may not know where it comes
from, but there's an enormous power at work.

—Christopher Reeve, *Still Me*

Write about what held you at gunpoint this week. Waiting for a
phone call with test results? Pain? A misunderstanding?

Write about the killer waiting in the basement. Write about terror.

Laura writes:
The doctor had called, had said he'd call back soon.
I hurried home to wait.
minutes and minutes, an eternity, more than an hour,
sitting in the sunlight of the open door.
Would the doctor really call back?
Had the bus brought Tim back from the field trip yet? Was he
waiting for me? Should I call someone else to take Melissa to her
ballet class?

But I couldn't use the phone, the doctor was supposed to call
    sitting in the sunlight in the open door, crying

Write a prayer or a petition. Write notes to God or to the gods or goddesses or to Buddha or to Jesus or To Whom It May Concern. Write for what you need.

Dave writes:
Teach me to taste the flavor of all I meet.

Teach me to know there is strength and harm to be borne, and how to bear.

Teach me to hear the silence within each, and let it still me.

Teach me to know the touch of another and feel it through.

Teach me to silence the noise of life and let life be clear.

Teach me to settle in and settle down and be comfortable here and now.

Teach me to be open and learn, not closed and stubborn.

Write what you need to learn.
Write about faith—having it or not having it.
Write about what the word faith means to you.
Write about your spiritual beliefs.

Susan writes: *Faith—more slippery than a fish pulled out of the water struggling for its life. When I was pulled out of my life by the hook of a brain tumor, I too was like the fish gasping for life. I found faith but it is elusive. It's not something I can hold onto with my will. So I went to church, was baptized, asked the deacons how to pray. I was too noisy—I found yoga and meditation. Yes, the quiet was a way to hear my faith. But gasping for air. That's not enough. You need guided visualizations, the relaxation response. But that's work! Guilt gets in the way of faith. Gasping for air.*

Neva writes: *I need my faith. When I pray I say 'Thy will, not mine be done' as a preface to my prayer. I try never to be dictating when I pray. I consult rather than delineate.*

Marilyn writes: *A friend went to the chapel at the hospital and promised to go to mass every day if I did well with my surgery. I feel guilty that she goes each morning. I tell her all is well now, she can relax, but she's afraid what might happen to me if she stops going.*

If you don't have spiritual beliefs, write about where and how you search for strength and meaning.

Write about one shining moment of happiness, one moment, brief and priceless.

8

LEAVING YOURSELF AT THE BORDER

But I'm a vegetarian, I keep saying like a mantra to all the doctors. I run four miles a day. I do yoga. I gave up smoking twenty years ago. Maybe I drink too much coffee and have a glass or two of wine every night, but I eat a lot of broccoli, I eat tofu. In fact, I eat more broccoli and tofu than anyone else I know. And I never ever get sick.

The hardest thing is to leave yourself, the innocent, healthy you that never before had to face her own mortality, at the border. That old relationship with your body, careless but friendly, taken for granted, suddenly ends. Your body becomes enemy territory. My left breast now belongs to my surgeon, and soon my oncologist and my radiation oncologist will stake their own claim to it. I'm grateful, so grateful, that I still have my breast, but it feels like a strange appendage to my body, numb and heavy, no longer mine. After the tubes and drain are taken out I look at it in the mirror—in spite of red welts of scars and rainbow-colored bruises, it's buoyed up by scar tissue and looks inappropriately perky compared to the healthy one.

There's a moment, not necessarily when you first hear your diagnosis, maybe weeks later, when you cross that border and know in your heart and soul that this is really serious. And this isn't where you belong.

That moment for me is when I walk through the door that says RADIATION ONCOLOGY. Both words are so foreign to me, so out of context with the rest of my life, that I could be landing on the moon.

The Ph.D. in Comp Lit, the years in Paris, the wall of books—you do not wear these badges on your johnny gown. No wonder I was forever giving our résumés to doctors and nurses, as if to beg them to see us for real, see what happy lives we had left at the border, which waited still like a dog on the front stoop.

—Paul Monette, *Borrowed Time, An AIDS Memoir*

A heart attack leaves you feeling that your most intimate friend has breached a fundamental trust. The body—bright youth, now tarnished and corrupted—loses its mind and violently assaults you, a monster within. You live thereafter with a strange sense of alienation.

—Lance Morrow, "Lessons of a Bad Heart," *Time* 3/19/01

Somewhere out there in that darkness are hundreds of thousands of women like myself, the new citizens of this other country, a huge army of the wounded, each believing herself to be alone in her shock and grief, with no target for her anger, no answering voice for her loss. In one moment of discovery, these lives have been transformed, just as mine has been, as surely as if they had been plucked from their native land and forced to survive in a hostile new landscape, fraught with dangers, real and imagined.

—Musa Mayer, *Examining Myself: One Woman's Story of Breast Cancer Treatment and Recovery*

At first, I was still afraid to join the ranks of cancer "victims." Support groups frightened me. I explained to my radiation oncologist, Dr. Charles Neal, that it depressed me to arrive at his waiting room and join those who were receiving radiation. I felt that I was entering the land of the dying. He said, "No, you are entering the place of hope— where the dying may be cured."

—Jerri Nielsen, M.D., *Ice Bound: A Doctor's Incredible Battle for Survival at the South Pole*

The sudden crossing over into illness or disability, becoming a patient, can feel like you're landing on another planet, or entering another country. What Susan Sontag calls "emigrating to the kingdom of the ill" in *Illness as Metaphor*.

Dave writes: *Crossing the border doesn't make one bicultural instantly. Joining a cancer support group, then leaving, thinking one will be more at home in one's faith support group, normal, cancer free—discovering, you returned a foreigner, in your own land. Home never the same on your side of the border, and not roots on the other—wanted or had. Border after border crossed until bicultural one becomes. Richness flows from each side, as you transfer from one to the other, always knowing the limits of each, and the gifts of both.*

Try making a metaphor out of this feeling; create your own country or planet. Think of it not in a literal way (i.e. the hospital) but as a nameless, imagined land you've never been to. Make up a geographical place with landscape and weather and customs. Is the air cold or hot? How does time work here? Do the clocks go faster than normal or get stuck at certain hours? Or do they melt like a Dali watch? What is used as currency—coins or food or sacrifices of some sort? What is the language like? What are the demands of this land? The regulations? The music and food and holidays?

Lou writes: *Oddly the sun shines constantly. There's no shade. Sometimes the clocks stop at two and don't move for weeks.*

If it's a planet you've landed on, what is the land made of? Cement? Silly Putty? Glue? What is gravity like? How does Earth look from your planet? What do you breathe and what do you eat? Are there other people on this planet?

By getting into metaphor you may come up with feelings and ideas you've never expressed before.

Maybe your geographical metaphor is closer to home.

Tippy writes, *Cancer is like living in California. You know there is the possibility of an earthquake. You experience the earthquake. Then live until the next earthquake occurs. Then there's the analysis. Is it the same earthquake, an aftershock? Or is it a new one?*

Caregivers also find themselves away from home, in a new place, missing the familiar.

Bob writes: *I really miss arguing . . . I miss a good old fashioned knock down—kiss and make-up argument. I hate the constipated feeling of letting little irritations build into resentment and boil into anger all bottled up inside. Why does this happen? It didn't before. But how can you argue with a cancer patient? I used to enjoy it, the juices flowed. But now I've lost the passion for it. No more righteous indignation as each trifling, momentary wrong is committed against me. Arguing with a cancer patient is like playing competitive chess with a six year old—can't get into it—doesn't seem right somehow. I still try every now and then, but with my right hand tied behind my back and my tongue muzzled so it won't spit any venom. The worst part is I never can win the argument—it's her ultimate trump card . . . It wasn't her fault—blame it all on chemo-brain.*

Write about what you miss. Write about what you took for granted.
Write about what you had to leave behind.

John writes what he left at the border: *Patience. The patience to wait her out. The patience to work it out. The patience to wait for my wife to return from her self-imposed exile—her self-protecting isolation, which leaves me so alone, hurt, muddled and angry. Time. It's all about time. It's time that we love. And I don't have the time.*

Judy writes: *Leaving behind the friends during my treatment who could/would not be with me. Who with fear of their own mortality felt so anxious for me, for themselves. For now I was the Judy who had cancer—would they catch some from me? The anxious and nosey who wanted blow by blow reports of my treatments—I avoided them. The transition of who I was to who I am now. The defining my borders—the saying no to them, fighting for my life. The not saying yes anymore to please them. The establishing even now of the me I have become, the moving forward, needing people in my life who see me as me and not the me as they wanted me to be. I left behind a lot of the person they thought I was. A newness, freshness, joy in living the now.*

9

FINAL STRAWS: PLASTIC BAGS
AND POLAROIDS

*T*he *waiting room of the radiation oncology department is filled with cancer* patients. No one looks well.

Then I remember that I too am a cancer patient.

I'm here today to be measured and tattooed. Radiation won't start until my incisions are healed. The room seems to hum and tick. I swear I can feel the radiation; there must be enough down here to blast us right out of Los Angeles County.

When my name is called I'm ushered into a changing room and given a plastic bag for my belongings. A sweet nurse named Tammy tells me to save the bag and keep it in the car so I can use it each time I come in for treatment. The idea of saving this one white plastic bag that says PATIENT'S BELONGINGS in big letters, bringing it back and forth from my car to the hospital five days a week for the five weeks of radiation treatment makes me feel crazy and rebellious— not at all a good patient but one who wants to use dozens, hundreds, the hospital's *entire supply* of plastic bags for my own selfish purposes.

I decide that I'll buy a very cool canvas bag instead of using the plastic one. I won't be removing a lot of clothes to haul around with me, just whipping off my top, that's all. It's like refusing to sit in those Naugahyde chairs half-naked before surgery—all of this feels so out of control, so lacking in dignity, that I grab at straws to get upset about. If I get really angry about the Big C, where will it lead? Where *can* it lead? Plastic bags are safer.

Since you can't go through radiation treatment twice on the same part of your body, the doctor tattoos black dots around my breast as a permanent marker of the perimeters of my treatment. I tell him that it would be very cool if he'd just tattoo some petals around the dots so they'd look like daisies instead of large blackheads.

I realize I'm obsessed with being cool. Maybe because cancer is so uncool.

The rainbow colors of my left breast have now faded into an alarming shade of yellow. My scars, the one under my arm for the lymph node dissection and the two-inch lumpectomy scar by the side of my nipple still look serious and raw.

A Polaroid is taken for my file—me and my yellow breast. The resulting photograph looks like it came from a trashy tabloid: "Scarred Yellow-Breasted Woman Found in Hospital Basement!" I look desperate in this photograph and not terribly sane.

The truth is, I love my legs, not for what they can do for me anymore, but simply because they are my legs. I look at my feet and see in their little spastic twitches an attempt to resolve the mystery of a nineteen-year-old trauma. They must see my body above the lesion as in a similar predicament. Calling down to them twitching and thrashing about . . . They must wonder about my life, just as I stare mystified at their sudden jerky movements. Are they in pain? . . . I feel them trying to tell me something. I am two personalities inhabiting one body, Siamese twins connected at the soul . . . Can my legs know I am still up here? They must. Whether they do or not, they are still mine. I wonder if they are lonely.

—John Hockenberry, Moving Violations

Everybody thinks cancer makes you thin. In fact, I'm getting fatter and fatter. I know this because people keep coming up to me and saying, "You look so well." Actually, I don't look particularly well—I'm pale and my hair is falling out behind my ears, as if I'm a failed street gang member whose zigzag shaving has gone wrong—so what they really mean is, "You look so fat."

—Ruth Picardie, *Before I Say Goodbye*

Life as a pilgrim on the road to AIDS is bittersweet. I've learned there is no straight line from hurt to healing . . . I've begun to think that, at the end of this road, as Elbert Hubbard once put it, "God will not look you over for medals, degrees, or diplomas, but for scars." Somewhere beneath the veneer of ordinary human vanity lurk the unconquerable fears and unmeasured regrets—the scars—that finally shape each pilgrim into something utterly unique, and utterly human. And this is, like it or not, God's purpose with us.

—Mary Fisher, *My Name Is Mary*

All the women in a book of photographs by Art Myers called *Winged Victory: Altered Images, Transcending Breast Cancer* are naked to the waist. They've all had mastectomies or lumpectomies, and some are posed with their spouse or partner, including Dora, who had her mastectomy sixty years ago.

At first the photographs are shocking, (women without breasts! women with huge scars!) and then, what's amazing is that they are not really shocking at all. They are simply photographs of women with only one breast, or none, or with scars on their breasts. There are quotes from each woman, and also from each lover.

What comes across is how beautiful the lover finds the woman. These are not the Polaroid shots in your file of you looking as if you were caught naked in the middle of a drug heist, but beautiful portraits of positive, dignified, gutsy, and, yes, sexy women.

One of the women in the book, Dani, writes: "One day, long before I met my sweetheart, Ralph, I stood naked in front of the mirror and made peace with the smooth mastectomy scar where my breast once was. I decided to feel truly beautiful . . ."

Write about deciding to feel a certain way about your body. Write about making peace with your body. Or write about not making peace with your body.

Carolyn writes: *My body has a different agenda than mine. I'm not used to this new relationship, feeling at odds with my body. I used to be the poster child for stunning health. Now I live in an alien's body that hurts . . . How do I honor a post-surgical body without it taking me hostage? Do I choose to fly forward in 5th gear again and just have these cancer checks as something in my schedule? The only other option is to whirrr in neutral. There can't be just two options; where's my continuum? Spock has taught me that there are always options. But this coin has only two sides. I'm going nowhere, flipping this coin. What else could my life be about, apart from this damn coin?*

Write about your body trying to take you hostage.
  Write about scars that show.
  Write about those that don't.
  Write about hiding scars, or not hiding them.

John writes: *People tell me scars show character. Yeah, I'm a character. But will I ever be able to view my cancer scars with distance and dispassion? The ones that don't show—these run much deeper. No superficial flesh wounds here. The ones we don't forget—the scars of a marriage failing.*

Laura, who's a professional storyteller, writes: *After the surgery I wrote a story—a modern fairy tale. When I tell this story I always end it with "And so that you know that my story is true, I have the scar to prove it." And then I point to the scar on my neck. I love my scar. Scars are tangible proof that we have healed.*

Susan writes: *The divots in my head are not mine, they belong to the tumor carved out by the surgeon. Do I need to own these too? Can I transform these scars into a connection with my soul, God?*

A student recently told me that my advice to just jump into a piece of writing, not to explain, but to get up close and personal right away, came to mind when a photographer friend advised her to always take two steps closer to whatever she was photographing.

With camera or pen, move in. Forget the background. Get up close. Reveal the truth. You don't need to write a whole lot of explanation—how, where, why, and who. Zoom in to what's important.

10

The Garish Colors of Craziness

*H*aving breast cancer taps into some not very attractive aspects of my character. One is my drama queen persona, which I realize is masquerading now as courage and openness. Another is a certain aura of specialness that I take on, rather like a halo. I am a *cancer patient*. And not just any old cancer, but *breast* cancer. *Newsweek's* cover-story cancer.

I tell everyone I have breast cancer, not just my family and friends, but all my students, the pet sitter, the guy who's putting a new roof on my house, members of my yoga class—and there's always this click of silence as they try to think of what to say, wondering what to do with this information. But how can I be brave and wonderful if no one knows I have this disease? Or rather, that I'm *battling* breast cancer, as the media always puts it. How can you run around with a great attitude if you keep the whole thing a secret?

R. spoils me the first few weeks. A saint: He gives up going into his office to hang out with me. He makes fresh orange juice and brings home sushi for supper, he goes to my doctor appointments with me. I tell him how grateful and blessed I am, how appreciated and loved he is. And then one day he comments on some small household task that needs to be done, suggesting that perhaps I could do it. I look at him in shock. "I have *cancer*," I say.

A critical illness is like a great permission, authorization or absolving.
It's all right for a threatened man to be romantic, even crazy, if he feels

like it. All your life you think you have to hold back your craziness, but when you're sick you can let it out in all its garish colors.

—Anatole Broyard, *Intoxicated by My Illness*

This is what I have to do so I can fall asleep. I put on my pajamas. But if it's cold, I wear long underwear, too. Sometimes gloves. Maybe even a hat. Make sure the sheets are perfectly flat. Line the blankets up precisely so there are no lumps. Put in earplugs so I won't be bothered by noise. Turn on the electric blanket, even in summer. Get into bed. Smooth out my pajamas (this takes quite some time). Do my rhythmic breathing.

—Louise DeSalvo, *Breathless, An Asthma Journal*

One thing I found that helped was that I never cried in front of my family. I discovered very quickly that if I had an emotional breakdown in front of them, I not only had to lift myself up, but I had to bring all of them up too.

So I just broke a window every day. Sometimes more than one a day. That really got rid of a big thing inside me . . . After a few weeks, the window repairman asked me why I was doing this. I told him I was really angry. He didn't ask me any more questions after that.

—Maria Smith, "A Broken Window Every Day," from *Inner Fire*

If you tend to shy away from acting strange or crazy in full view of others, if you want to protect your windows and other fragile objects from your rage, the place you can let it all hang out is in your writing.

Members of the workshop write about their cancer patient badge, caregiver's halo, their rage. Margie writes about trying to get the plumber to come to her house. *Should I play the chemo card? As in, I'm having chemo tomorrow and I really need you to come today.* When she reads this out loud, Dave says, "Don't mention the chemo! He'll make you pay cash!" And they both hoot with laughter.

Feeling deep pain and grief and fear doesn't preclude other, often contradictory, emotions. As my yoga teacher says, "You can't hold the pose perfectly; you're human. It's okay to wobble."

When you wobble, fall out of your pose, take off your mask, what do you do?

Suzanne says she feels it's not socially acceptable to air her rage unless it's on paper. John (who's wearing a T-shirt with the words: "You Didn't Think I Chose This Look Did You?" printed on the front, and "Hair By Chemo" on the back) holds up his fist and says, "Rage on, girl!"

She writes: *I'm angry that I have cancer, that I had chemo, radiation, lumpectomy, mastectomy, prophylactic mastectomy, reconstruction, and oophorectomy. I'm angry that all the above HURT. I'm angry that my children don't understand why mommy is sick so much, that I can't swoop them up in my arms and swing them around and around . . . I'm angry that I don't like people. They smell, they are noisy, take up space, eat more than their share, snore, fart, judge, scowl, disapprove. I'm angry that being human has never been good enough for me . . . I'm angry that the children drop chocolate chips, mud, popcorn, pudding, spaghetti and juice on my carpet . . .*

Write about your anger. Air it all out on the page. Write about the colors of your craziness. Write about your halo or badge. Write about the strangest thing you've done recently.

Let yourself wobble. Take off the mask. Write what's underneath.

11

SNAKE OIL PROMISES

W<small>*hen you get a major disease there's suddenly a lot to read. I read all 610*</small> pages of *Dr. Susan Love's Breast Book* and also books about self-healing, the immune system, alternative medicine. Some of this makes sense, and I wonder if my immune system crashed and burned during the six years I lost both of my parents and went through a divorce. Weirdly, the tumor was right over my heart. On the other hand, if you get cancer because you go through loss and a bad time, wouldn't everyone over the age of thirty have cancer? Who on this planet doesn't go through losses and bad times? But maybe we all have these vulnerable spots in our bodies, and that's where something breaks down—whether with cancer or something else.

In one book I read about "needing" my illness—a concept that I find peculiar at best.

In another I read the profile of a cancer patient. According to this theory, all my life I have been restricted in expressing emotion and have practiced self-denial. I have been too kind, which is why I now have breast cancer. I read this aloud to R. and he laughs.

"Is it *that* funny?" I ask.

"Yes," he says.

The truth is I have never allowed an emotion to go unexpressed—an aspect of my personality that's often unappreciated by my family and close friends. And I'm not very good at self-denial. I know how to say No; I can be selfish. But what if I *had* been a saint? What if I'd practiced self-denial and more control over my emotions, how would I feel reading this stuff? Really furious, I think. *You tried to be so good and look what it got you—cancer.*

I want to believe that an upbeat attitude will keep my immune system perking away so that cancer won't spread or come back. But a few of the healing books make me angry. The ones that say cancer patients are empty of feeling and have no sense of self, the ones that explain your childhood with psychobabble. The books, full of snake oil promises, that preach that you can cure whatever disease you have with the right attitude.

What does this mean? That if we die we haven't tried hard enough, that somehow we've caused our own death out of laziness? That those of us who die are losers?

I want to believe that there's something I can do to make all this turn out right.

But all I believe in for sure is laughter, the way it makes my body feel—as if music is running through my veins and my skin is humming. I believe in the power of words and art and music to heal and calm my soul. I believe that eating a lot of pasta, olive oil, and garlic, practicing yoga, and running on the beach make my body happy and healthy. I believe that animals and nature offer comfort and solace and are as close as you can get to God. I believe in hanging out with my family and friends, loving them with all my heart and being loved back. I believe it doesn't hurt to pray.

I don't believe for one instant that I needed or created or deserved this disease.

"You create your own health," the teacher is saying. Obediently, we will now vomit up the detritus of our former lives, so that we may be full of radiant health and pain free. We will now choose a mantra, as commanded. Two syllables, like a healthy heartbeat. I believe in none of this, but would like to believe in meditation and breathing. I am filled with both longing to believe and adolescent contempt for it, so my

mantra for today is fuck you. *I'd like to take the fluffy-haired teacher, before whom I lie supplicant in my usual position, and make her suffer her own lie of responsibility for physical health, for control over the body's frailty. You with the perfect mobility, say that lie over and over to the young stroke victims whose heads wobble like toy birds, as they lose, forever, their real youth in this rehabilitation hospital.*

—Suzanne E. Berger, *Horizontal Woman*

Over lunch today, an old friend asked me in all seriousness whether I thought I had a "cancer personality." What would that be? Someone who holds anger in, she said. She's been on antidepressants for over a year, and I have the cancer personality?

—Peggy Orenstein, "Breast Cancer at 35,"
New York Times Magazine 6/19/97

The arrogance which says I alone bear the responsibility for my body, for my fate, can suspend compassion. What are we to do, holding these tenets, when people we love fail to stay healthy? What if we "fail" to be well ourselves; mustn't that be a moral or spiritual failure? And if we ask for what we get, if all our suffering and illnesses are brought upon ourselves—cancer from repressed anger, AIDS from wounded sexuality—then what is the role of compassion? . . . We trivialize pain if we regard it as a preventable condition the spirit need not suffer. If we attempt to edit it out, will it away, regard it as our own reaction, then don't we erase some essential part of the spirit's education? Pain is one of our teachers, albeit our darkest and most demanding one.

—Mark Doty, *Heaven's Coast*

In the movie *Bull Durham*, there's a scene in which Kevin Costner tells Susan Sarandon what he believes in. The most famous line is about his belief in "long, slow, deep, soft wet kisses that last three days." Other beliefs he holds include Lee Harvey Oswald acted alone and opening your presents Christmas morning rather than Christmas Eve. He also lists things he believes should be outlawed, such as Astroturf and the designated hitter.

What do you believe in? Write for ten minutes. Fling down everything that comes into your mind—spiritual beliefs, political opinions, what matters most in life, what you believe is good for your body and your soul, how to raise kids, how holidays should be celebrated, the quirky beliefs that you usually don't talk about—

Deb writes: *I believe dogs are angels. That they were sent down with fur instead of wings. And they watch over you. And never judge you. You can walk around naked, with your pudgy gut sticking out, and they don't care. You can wear stripes with plaids, so what? You can be messy, angry, stupid, lazy, not funny and so uncool, and they still want to sit next to you. Your feet can stink, they love you even more. I believe in this unconditional love. But I don't believe it can happen between two people.*

What do you believe about love? About friendship, about families, about animals?

Neva writes: *I believe in love, in caring, in nurturing, in satisfying sex, in enjoying each minute as it comes.*

Jean writes: *I believe that telling the truth is dangerous. I believe we're all much more afraid than we pretend to be. I believe the words we say and the way we act can change and mutate but the bedrock of what we believe stays the same.*

What myths surround your physical condition? What do you believe about your body? Your health?

Dave writes:
I believe life is to be understood and remain a mystery.
I believe each of us lives our own misunderstandings, mysteries and understandings.
I believe in misunderstandings becoming mysteries on the way to understandings.

Cancer is a fact.
Surrounded by my hopes and fears and all sorts of misunderstandings.
It becomes a mystery until one understands what one can.

I don't know how or why some get cancer and others don't.
I don't know how and why some survive and others don't.
I hope I didn't do anything to get cancer,
yet can do something not to have it recur.

I believe in acting true to my beliefs,
and living through my misunderstandings,
through mystery, to grain after grain of understanding and belief.

Write about what you don't believe in.
Write about what you wish you could believe in.

12

INWARD BOUND

I go to a networking meeting. The women who attend are all in different phases of breast cancer. We're supposed to have an upbeat attitude, and God knows I am trying to be upbeat.

We sit in a cozy room—nine women with breast cancer, a guest speaker, and a therapist. When it's my turn to introduce myself I tell them how my fiancé found the lump, how the tumor didn't show up on the mammogram, that I just had a lumpectomy, that I'm about to start radiation, and I'm waiting to find out if I have to have chemo. Then I do a short riff on how healthy I am and how utterly amazing and shocking all this is to me. I speak in a cheery, upbeat sort of voice.

A beautiful woman in a wheelchair whose cancer has spread to her bones is very dignified and calm as she introduces herself and talks about her chances of survival. Another woman says that her cancer has come back in the other breast, and she cries. Another is starting chemo this week; she cries too. We talk about soy and tofu and flax seed oil. Where to buy it, how to fix it, what to do with it. The guest speaker talks about retreats, groups of women going off together and doing risky, difficult physical things like scaling mountains and hanging from trees. Kind of an Outward Bound for women with breast cancer. This isn't something I'd want to do with or without breast cancer.

On the way home I stop at the health food market and buy soy milk, powdered soy, flax seed oil, firm tofu, silky tofu, pounds of organic vegetables. As I drive toward R.'s house I start to cry. I've just bought bags of *cancer food*. I'm somebody who has to eat special food, *cancer food*. Then I think of the woman in the wheelchair, the woman starting chemo, the one who just found a new lump, and feel guilty for being upset about *just food* for God's sake. But feeling guilty makes me cry even harder.

And I face the truth: I am not upbeat. I've got a real shitty attitude.

. . . Dr. Khanjani thinks that within six months I should be well. So it's worth it to eat almost nothing that I really like, although last night I had an excellent supper which consisted of a small piece of flounder, broiled with just a touch of olive oil and paprika on it; brown rice mixed with very small peas that come in a can (I shouldn't have done that, but they did taste delicious!); half an avocado, on which I squeezed some lemon juice; and then, most delicious, an apple baked with honey and cinnamon. So that was a real feast and I have nothing to complain about.
—May Sarton, *After the Stroke, A Journal*

And one day, lo and behold, my little ninety-five pound body started to get hungry. I hadn't really eaten in over a month . . .

I started to want things from my childhood that I hadn't thought of in years. I wanted French toast . . . Suddenly food was all I could think about. I wanted oatmeal and brown sugar. I wanted pancakes with bacon and syrup. I wanted bagels with cream cheese. Somehow as my taste buds came back, they came back for foods of my childhood, things that were in the fridge and the cupboards when I was little—Cameo cookies, Muenster cheese, sour cream. Gene and Grace were always going to the supermarket—I kept coming up with new cravings. It got so Gene and Grace wouldn't mention food around me. Hot dogs—I wanted hot dogs with mustard and relish and everything . . . doughnuts and crispy French fries . . . horrible foods, stuff that you would never eat because it would give you cancer. Everything I wanted was stuff that the American Cancer Society said, "Don't eat this—it will give you cancer." . . .

—Gilda Radner, *It's Always Something*

When you write about food you get into specific, concrete detail right away. All of our senses are engaged, we have memories about mealtimes and favorite dishes growing up, we all have something to say about it. And most of us have a certain amount of emotional baggage about food. How and where and what and with whom we eat is never trivial or meaningless.

Write about food—the best meal you had this week. The worst.

Write about eating too much.

Write about not being able to eat. Write about not having an appetite. Write about being nauseated.

Bob writes: *My more recent progress in life has come when I open my mind and stop doing things on automatic. Food is automatic—usually—and that makes it uneventful. But the feeling of selecting, smelling, tasting and swallowing—ripe strawberries come to mind—again until full, then liking the feeling and proceeding beyond reason to past full to uncomfortable—*

Write about what you had for breakfast on winter mornings when you were in grade school. What you brought in your lunch box to school or what the school cafeteria served.

Emily writes: *I hate oatmeal. I have always hated oatmeal. And I always will hate oatmeal. But oatmeal, I discovered when I was very young, has curious properties, ephemeral properties, properties—that before the "couldn't be's" set in—are the fuel of intrigue. The grown-ups had long departed, bored sitting there, staring me down. "Sit there until the oatmeal is gone, Emily."*

Write about a restaurant you love.

Write about comfort food.

Maura writes: *Food is not easy to write about in five minutes. Providing meals is something my family expects me to do. My nineteen-year-old son stayed home from college to care for me and yet would ask every night, "When is dinner?" Sometimes I wanted to scream—"You can see I can't even open my eyes for ten consecutive minutes. How can you expect me to provide dinner for six, including your girlfriend!" A cancer diagnosis does not erase years of being expected to be the caretaker. My comfort food is whatever my friends bring me to eat.*

If you're alone do you graze at the kitchen counter, or do you get takeout and watch television? Or do you set the table for yourself and serve a meal in the same way you would if someone were with you? Does someone deliver your dinner to your house, or does it come on a hospital tray to your room?

If you eat with someone, what is the conversation about? What is the room you're eating in like? Are there rituals?

Or, if you're unable to eat, write about that. Write about one thing that tastes good to you.

Write about what you crave.

13

TIED TO RAILROAD TRACKS

M_y *left arm still feels sore and stiff. I walk the wall with my fingers, an* exercise you're supposed to do three times a day. Fear fades in and out like static.

Tomorrow I see the oncologist and this is my plan: If the news isn't good, if the tumor is aggressive and I need chemotherapy, I will go immediately to a bookstore after the doctor's visit and buy as many books—novels, poetry, essays—maybe CDs too, as I want; my Visa card will melt under the book binge I intend to carry out. Afterward I'll come home to my own house in Hermosa Beach, put on a Mozart piano concerto, and call R., who's out of town on business, then Nicki, Sally, Ruth, and all the rest of my friends, and then I'll read. For once in my life I'll have a really good excuse just to sit around the house and do nothing but read.

Later I'll go out and buy a wig and a turban, and some really gorgeous clothes.

I keep coming back to clothes. This is so odd. In real life I never care about my clothes—all my clothes are black because I don't like to shop, and if you just wear one color, it simplifies things. But now I'm thinking black looks so serious, so funeral-like.

I make a list of all the stuff I'll buy. Saving money at this point seems to be, well, optimistic at best.

And then I think—this is such a joke. Here I am trying to control things. Thinking that buying books and clothes will somehow contain my feelings, make everything okay. It's like planning and making a list while strapped to the railroad tracks with the train coming right at you.

The design for my future is on slides in the pathology department at the hospital. I have no control over any of this, and that's what really makes me crazy.

❦

Luckily, there is a third therapeutic strategy which I am developing almost single-handedly, though sadly not in a controlled trial situation at present, so fellow patients will have to find their own precious path. Essentially, after months of careful research, I have discovered a treatment that is a) cheapter than complementary therapy, b) a hell of a lot more fun than chemotherapy, and c) most important, incredibly effective! Retail therapy! By this, I mean personal indulgence or escapism of any kind.

—Ruth Picardie, *Before I Say Goodbye*

. . . I began to do a lot of shopping in a store called Laise Adzer in Beverly Hills. It has Moroccan-style women's clothing—lots of cotton with fringe. It also has scarves you can wrap around your head, and turbans are shown with all the clothes. I realized that if I just bought clothes like that and dressed that way, I could wear scarves around my head. That would hide my baldness. I bought a whole bunch of scarves and a couple of outfits that I could wear if I got invited somewhere. . . . The happier I was, the more I piled on my head. I dressed like a harem girl. At last I had found a character in which I could come back into the social world.

—Gilda Radner, *It's Always Something*

When you're ill you instinctively fear a diminishment and disfigurement of yourself. It's that, more than dying, that frightens you. You're going to become a monster. I think you have to develop a style when you're ill to keep from falling out of love with yourself. It's important to stay in love with yourself. That's known as the will to live. And your style is the instrument of your vanity. If they can afford it, I think it would be good therapy, good body narcissism, for cancer patients to buy a whole new wardrobe, mostly elegant, casual clothes.

—Anatole Broyard, *Intoxicated by My Illness*

Write about the character in which you can return to your old life. What kind of style can you assume? How are you going to stay in love with yourself?

Susan writes: *I could buy a house and redecorate it. I really want to have a home. I want to put roots down. A puppy too, yes, that would be my style . . . I want to plant my roots with others in the same old clothes I have. I want to wear the same clothes every day.*

Candy writes: *I want to appear normal but I guess when I look around the room—what exactly is normal? I am into baseball caps now and never in my life have I worn them. But my life is different now so I make these baseball caps a little fancier.*

During the most difficult times, right after your diagnosis, waiting for test results, being in pain—it's often hard to concentrate. Sometimes all you can manage is a list, or to jot down random thoughts without following them through. In a poem entitled "His Bathrobe Pockets Stuffed with Notes," Raymond Carver lists random memories, ideas for work, observations, and quotes from both the famous and not famous. If you were to stuff the pockets of your bathrobe with notes, what quotes, memories, ideas, observations would be written on them?

Make a list of what you have control over. Another list of what you can't control.

Make a list of what you need—more clothes, or love, or whatever. Then a list of what you have.

Laura lists:

I need more love.	*I have too many people loving me.*
I need six more decades.	*I have this moment.*
I need a future.	*I have now.*
I need air.	*I have the ability to breathe.*
I need to begin again.	*I have confusion as to where to start.*
I need fewer needs.	*I have more than I need.*

Make a list of things you can't do. Make another of things you can do.

Carlie writes: *I can't touch the stars, but I can accept the sky.*

Make a list of ways in which you can nurture yourself.

Make a list of topics you want to make lists about.

Fill your pockets with notes.

14

AMPUTATING THE WRONG LIMB

There's a big sign on the door to the oncology office that says Cancer Care Associates. You'd think they could use a euphemism—maybe Creative Care, or better yet, Constant Care.

My two daughters, who have left work to come with me for this appointment since R. is still out of town, seem larger than anyone else in the waiting room. They're so healthy and beautiful, they exude so much energy and life.

Terrified about this first appointment with the oncologist, I sit between them, feeling their warmth, smelling their clean shampoo smell, wanting to soak up their health and energy and clear thinking. I feel so much love for my girls that my heart hurts whenever I look at them. I worry; what does my breast cancer bode for their own health?

The room is filled with people who have no hair, people who are frail and ill; this is where you come for chemotherapy treatments. Even the family members and friends who are with the patients seem frail, older. There are baskets of hard candies and free cans of Ensure. Serious magazines and brochures.

It's like the waiting room in radiation oncology. I feel out of place here. I don't feel like a person who has cancer. It suddenly occurs to me that maybe I don't really have cancer. Maybe the hospital has made a terrible mistake. You hear about this all the time—slides get mixed up, unbelievable errors are made. I've read newspaper reports of doctors even amputating the wrong leg.

This, of course, would explain everything. They put the wrong report in my file! The pathology report of my *benign* tumor is in someone else's file! This would explain why I feel so out of place as a cancer patient. Quickly I decide how magnanimous I'll be when the hospital discovers their huge mistake; I won't sue.

When we're ushered into the examining room to meet the oncologist, my fantasy fades. I'm simply going crazy, that's all. There's my chart; it's getting fat—so many tests and so many doctors. No mistakes possible. In the months to come, I'll realize and understand that going crazy when you visit your doctor is perfectly normal for cancer patients. Once you've heard the unthinkable, you know it's possible to hear it again, or worse.

The oncologist is very low-key and smart. I can see my girls relax; they trust him and no doubt find him attractive. Asian-American, in his late thirties, he's wearing khaki pants that are beautifully pressed and a collarless blue shirt. He's very lean, and his hair has been buzzed down almost clear to his scalp. ("To make his bald chemo patients feel more comfortable," one of my daughters will comment later.)

He gets right to the point. "You don't need chemotherapy," he says. I feel myself dissolve in relief, teary and grateful.

"I'm even on the fence about you taking tamoxifen," he says.

That's good because I don't want to take tamoxifen, the drug that acts like a bouncer at the door of your breast cells. It blocks estrogen in your breast, while apparently acting like estrogen itself in other parts of your body. Even Dr. Love says this is a very peculiar drug.

I've been hatching a new theory; the reason I have breast cancer is because I was on hormone therapy for the past ten years—prescribed by a male doctor. I can climb on my feminist soap box about this. It makes me angry that I was on estrogen for that long, but this also offers a neat cause and effect that makes me feel better. Getting breast cancer wasn't just wild and unfathomable chance, there was a scientific reason with political implications.

I don't want any more doctors fooling around with my hormones. Though I'm not sure my own theory even makes sense; the bottom line is I just don't want any more drugs. I ask the doctor about alternative medicine and diet.

He hedges, talks about quality of life. "I've seen patients with negative attitudes and terrible eating habits who survive," he says, and then adds, "People need the sense that they have some control."

And all the time as a background of pain and terror and disbelief, a thin high voice was screaming that none of this was true, it was all a bad dream that would go away if I became totally inert. Another part of me flew like a big bird to the ceiling of whatever place I was in, observing my actions and providing a running commentary, complete with suggestions of factors forgotten, new possibilities of movement, and ribald remarks. I felt as if I was always listening to a concert of voices from inside myself, all with something slightly different to say, all of which were quite insistent and none of which would let me rest.
                        —Audre Lorde, *The Cancer Journals*

I was still in denial, still thinking, There's been a big mistake here. Any minute someone's going to come in and say, "Sorry, wrong person; they meant somebody down the hall. It's not you. You're free to go."
                        —Christopher Reeve, *Still Me*

I still have such conflicted feelings about hiding the diagnosis. What's privacy and what's denial? How much is guilt and the lingering self-hatred of the closet? I've tried to fever-chart the stages as they evolved over the next six months, but the simplest way to put it is that Roger fought his way back to real life, and I fell completely apart.
                        —Paul Monette, *Borrowed Time, An AIDS Memoir*

Start with the words: This is all a bad dream . . . and write for five minutes.

Write the ways in which you deny what's happening with your body. Or your loved one's body.

Tippy writes: *I'm not sure I was ever in denial about the fact of George's cancer, but I was on the seriousness of it. (Duh. Weren't you listening? Haven't you heard the expression* serious as cancer?) *Well, most boo-boos could be fixed. You operate, get chemo, radiation. Voila. All done. I heard the news announcement that those with lung cancer who continue to smoke can get a brain tumor. I passed on the info and poof the info disappeared into the ether. Merrily we roll along, roll a long—until the next time. Merrily . . . until the next time. Until the brick wall.*

Write about the brick wall in your life.

Write about a visit you've had recently with the doctor. Try writing it in the third person. Sometimes when you write about *he* or *she* instead of *I* there's more distance, a slightly different view.

Write about the strangest, weirdest theory you've had about your illness or accident.

Start with the words *There's been a mistake . . .* and write for five minutes.

15

ONE CELL GOING NUTS

A few days later I pick up my records and slides from the hospital to deliver to UCLA Medical Center for my second opinion exam next week. Before driving to Westwood, I sit in the parking lot and read my records.

Up until now I've imagined cancer as this one little cell going nuts. It had a cartoon quality to it—all the *splats* and *pows* weren't quite real, it was the boulder that temporarily flattens Mr. Coyote. But there's nothing cartoonish about my records; this is serious business.

The ultrasound found: "9mm × 7mm lobular solid mass with somewhat angular margins in the left breast at 3 o'clock."

The pathologist report found: "Invasive grade III/III carcinoma. 1 cm nodule, extending to the outer surgical margin. Eight negative lymph nodes. Relatively favorable biomarkers with the exception of ploidy and HER2. ER and PR positive."

The oncologist writes that my chances estimated for a five-year survival rate disease free are in the mid-eighty range. The odds go up a few percentage points if I take tamoxifen.

Relatively favorable biomarkers? With the *exception* of ploidy and HER2? And what, please, is *ploidy*? It sounds like something ill-fitting pants would be made of; some terrible, sleazy material.

I want better odds, I want some guarantees here. I want someone to recognize that my maternal grandmother and great-grandmother died in their nineties and factor that in. That my mother died *early* at eighty-seven. That my father believed, when he was eighty-six, he was dying much too young.

That evening I read up on what I found in my records. I realize how unequipped I am to understand this enough to make wise decisions. Is it better just to trust your doctors and not read this? How educated can you get reading a few books and searching the Internet? How do you handle the contradictions?

I feel lost in the words of my own medical records. I have become a generic patient, I am a case, another statistic. I am a "well appearing woman in no acute distress," according to my records.

These are my records, but where is my story? Where are the details of who I am, the particulars of my life?

> i was leaving my fifty-eighth year
> when a thumb of ice
> stamped itself hard near my heart
>
> you have your own story
> you know about the fear the tears
> the scar of disbelief
>
> you know that the saddest lies
> are the ones we tell ourselves
> you know how dangerous it is
>
> to be born with breasts
> you know how dangerous it is
> to wear dark skin
>
> i was leaving my fifty-eighth year
> when I woke into the winter
> of a cold and mortal body
>
> thin icicles hanging off
> the one mad nipple weeping

have we not been good children
did we not inherit the earth

but you must know all about this
from your own shivering life
    —Lucille Clifton "1994,"
        Living on the Margins,
    Women Writers on Breast Cancer

. . . *for all the astonishing technical advances of the twentieth century, we still possess an unquenchable instinct to make ourselves part of a story. It's this that makes us human. Yet talk to any doctor in this vein and they will pooh-pooh such suggestions. Large or small, a stroke, they will say, is no more than the smallest physical malfunction, a wonky configuration of blood in a cerebral artery . . .*
    —Robert McCrum, *My Year Off, Recovering Life After a Stroke*

I thought of how it had felt to read the pathology report after my mastectomy, and see my breast described as "the specimen received," covered by an "ellipse of tan soft skin measuring 24 × 8 cm." I thought of a late medieval painting I'd seen once of one of the Catholic martyrs, bearing her severed breasts on a platter as a grotesque offering of piety.
    —Musa Mayer, *Examining Myself: One Woman's Story of Breast*
                Cancer Treatment and Recovery

Like campers huddled around a fire, we were mesmerized by T-cell lore. The moral of every story seemed to be the same: one had to unhitch himself from statistics, had to be greater than the sum of his cells. The protagonists of some tales were healthy while others were ill, but each had found a way to face the future, either by surrendering to, or raging against, uncertainty.

    —Bernard Cooper, *Truth Serum*

The poet, William Carlos Williams, who was also a physician, gave this advice to Robert Coles when he was in medical school: "Their story, yours, mine—it's what we all carry with us on this trip we take, and we owe it to each other to respect our stories and learn from them."

As patients, we are still individuals who are living unique stories no matter what our circumstances. Writing helps us discover our story.

You don't have to write the story of your life, your accident, your illness, your heartbreak, from beginning to end in a long, linear fashion, culminating with illumination. You can start in the middle, or in the present. Or jump around and not know where it's going.

Think of looking through a window at a specific time in your life—what does the landscape or the room look like from this angle? What's the weather like? Who can you see through this window? What words do you hear? Take quick views through the windows. Write for five minutes at a time.

Or think of writing squares of a quilt. You don't have to write the whole quilt, just small squares, one by one. Later you can stitch it all together.

Nancy writes:

This year as I look at my Passover table ablaze with candles, I will see the Seder plate with its ceremonial foods. Only this year I give my own interpretation:

A roasted egg—for new life
Bitter herbs—for irony
Salted water—for tears
Matzoh—the gift of life
Apples, honey and nuts—for serendipity
Wine—for life's joys
A family gathered—for love

Passover—almost a year since I was diagnosed. Moses led the chosen from bondage to wander in the desert, and find the Promised Land. Has it only been one year? It seems like forty.

To life! L'chayim!

Laura writes: *Well, I cannot write about my childhood—the canned raviolis when I was home sick or all the meals I was not fed. So many memories are more bitter than sweet. My mother, paranoid schizophrenic, trained us, brainwashed us to remember the bad. She commemorates the anniversary of every horrible event—the day her grandfather molested her; the day she and her mother plotted to kill him; the day my father left; the day he refused to hold her hand in church; the day she was admitted to the mental hospital for the 2nd time. Fuck memories! . . . The window is closed.*

Margie brings her eighty-five-year-old mother, Fannie, who is visiting from the Midwest, to the workshop. Fannie tells me she wants to write about her life but is overwhelmed by the idea and doesn't know where to begin. We talk about writing her story scene by scene, as if looking through small windows or making squares of a quilt, without the need to go from beginning to now. Fannie embarks on this project with great energy and enthusiasm—and eventually comes up with over a hundred pages of lively and interesting stories about her life.

Later she tells me that one day she was frustrated when she couldn't remember the name of the woman who introduced her to her future husband. The next time she sat down to write, the name *Dorothy* popped into her head, the name she'd been trying to think of. She said she'd never have remembered the name if she hadn't been writing about the past.

I loved hearing this because it illustrates the idea that everything we need to tell our story, and to be creative—our memories and fantasies and ideas—is in us, available, waiting to be drawn out. It's a deep well within you. You don't need to measure the water or the depth, just trust that it's all down there. Your job is to write, to give it a voice.

Think of a small window into your own life. A birthday party when you were in grade school. Buying a new pair of shoes. Your grandmother cooking a favorite family recipe. A beloved pet. The first time you fell in love. Your mother's face. Your father's voice.

Keep looking through the windows. If it's painful, keep writing.

If the thought that this might be boring and not worth the time or effort ever crosses your mind, think how you'd feel if you discovered that a great grandparent had written down all the stories and details, all the thoughts and feelings of his or her life; how priceless those pages would be to you.

When Fannie died a year after she came to the workshop, Margie wrote to me about the difference writing had made in her mother's life, and added, "Her memoirs are a gift to our family for generations to come."

16

DANCING IN FRONT OF
CHRISTMAS TREES

*D*r. *Susan Love is no longer director of the UCLA/Revlon Breast Center,* but she's left her mark. None of this plastic bag filled with your clothes nonsense, no sitting around in public half-naked in a jonny gown. You're given a room and they—the doctors!—come to you. The psychologist, the radiation oncologist, the surgeon, the oncologist all file through as if you're granting celebrity interviews. They even give R. and me a little tape machine so we can record it all.

I'm heavily into my star patient routine—I want to be the fastest recovered, the most psychologically sound, the happiest and healthiest and most amazing patient they've ever seen. I remember a home movie that my father took the first Christmas my baby brother was born. I was five years old and dancing madly in front of the Christmas tree, desperate; I wanted all the attention, I wanted to be the star.

And here I am fifty years later, still dancing.

I tell each doctor who passes through that R. found the lump and here he is, my fiancé, the star lump finder. In between interviews and exams, R. says, "Maybe I have a future career in this sort of thing. You know, an odd kind of talent, checking breasts."

"In your dreams," I say.

The third day the lady from the American Cancer Society visits with her toys: a short rope, a rubber ball, cotton pads to stuff in my bra. I am bright and perky, I am cooperative and funny, I am the good girl

student. I sit cross-legged on my bed, my dirty hair pulled into a ponytail, in rapt attention, nodding pleasantly at everything. I am utterly stupid, of course; an hour after she leaves I realize I am the mastectomy patient she was talking about.

—Annette Williams Jaffee, "The Good Mother," from
Living on the Margins, Women Writers on Breast Cancer

The patient is the star of the show, but the audience varies: lame-duck specialists; ghouls; true friends; compassion junkies; hypochondriacs; and people who welcome the chance to address a captive audience. (It intrigued me to see the relief on my friends' faces when, as one put it, they discovered that 'you are not a drooling vegetable.')

—Robert McCrum, *My Year Off, Recovering Life After a Stroke*

People weren't interested in playing extras in my melodrama. They wanted a key supporting role in a near-death experience. The more I sought meaning in the little details of my new life, the more the people around me thought I was nuts. "Move on with your life," they said. But my life wouldn't budge, and there were steps everywhere.

—John Hockenberry, *Moving Violations*

Write about what kind of patient or caregiver you are. Are you cranky? Or are you dancing madly? Are you a tough girl or good guy? Demanding or quiet? Write for five minutes.

Write about what kind of a patient or caregiver you would like to be.

Marilyn writes about going into surgery for a brain tumor and coming on to her surgeon: *Terrified, I wanted him to like me and to care if I survived! Maybe it was the drugs. I told him I loved him. He smiled and got closer to my face to see if I understood him. I looked him in the eyes, then puckered up my lips . . . 'Kissy, Kissy, Kissy.' He laughed. In fact laughter grew as I continued my comments to the doctor. I have no mem-*

ory of the following remarks I made . . . One only need use their imagination. I never asked.

Jean writes: *I want my doctors and nurses to love me and care for me. To see me as sweet and good, to look forward to my appointments. I want even the receptionist to like me. I figure if they love me, I'll get more of what I want, more of what I need, a better chance to be healthy. I think medical care administered in a more loving manner is more effective.*

Beatrice writes about being a caregiver in the third person: *Boy, were they surprised. The girl who would never settle down, never compromise, never give up her freedom, and never change dirty diapers for any amount of money . . . she was really good at this caretaker bit. . . . Where did all this love and patience come from? Where had all the squeamish selfishness gone? How could she make this sacrifice, they asked. What she marveled at is how it had given her the greatest gift—the sense of having done something worthwhile—of having given meaning to her life. Finally she was good at something that mattered, something no one else could or would do for her mother.*

17

Cancer Is Not a Car

You can dance around a lot and joke, but there's always 3:00 A.M., the midnight of your soul, the dark tunnel to get through. No matter how loving your family and friends, no one truly understands what it's like except for people going through that same dark tunnel.

I feel the need to be with people who are going through the same thing I am, women who have just found out they have breast cancer. So in April I sign up at The Wellness Community to join the newly diagnosed breast cancer support group.

Once on NPR I heard a guy putting down support groups. He said if he had car problems, he wouldn't want to hang out with a group of people who also had car problems—he'd want to find someone who could fix his car and hang out with that person. I figure there are huge differences between cancer and cars. Also, I've read that the survival rate for women with breast cancer is higher for those who are in support groups.

My friend Ruth works at The Wellness Community in Redondo Beach, and I'd been planning for over a year to volunteer there to conduct a writing workshop. I'm glad it didn't work out; in my mind I had thought of the people going there as *them*. They were *the other*. They had *cancer*. And now I am one of them; I too am the other. If I had gone there before getting cancer, I think I might have conducted a workshop in a cautious, polite, rather sickening way.

The first woman I meet in the group, Beth, is about the same age as my daughters. She's a physical therapist, tall and very chic, with a turban wrapped around her head; she's already started chemo and has lost her hair. She's in her *early thirties*; how can someone this young have breast cancer?

Then there's Polly, who's thirty-nine, divorced, an actress with three children. Dee, just turned forty, works for an ad agency and lives alone. Three others are in their forties; Carol, Asian, with a family and a job, Betty, a clinical audiologist who lives with her boyfriend and flies to Mexico on weekends to do free hearing clinics, and Elana, who is divorced and angry about absolutely everything. Doris, in her early fifties, also lives alone and hasn't had any treatment yet. And Sandra, British, around my age, married with kids and grandchildren.

Immediately this feels better than that networking meeting I went to. Here, we're all in the same boat, all of us had been going along with our lives when suddenly, within the past month or two, each of us learned we had breast cancer. We're all in shock, all amazed and angry and scared. When it's my turn, I introduce myself with my usual riff—R.'s discovery of the lump (which is now assuming mythic proportions in my tale), my treatment so far, and then how shocking and out of context all this is for me. The response of this group is more like a Southern Baptist church: Amen to that, sister. Amen.

We're all in this boat together, trying to ride out the storm.

Or to mix metaphors, if we all have broken cars, at least they were all broken at the same time.

Dee talks about having a baseline mammogram when she turned forty and finding out she had cancer, how she's somebody who runs and rides her bike at the beach, not somebody who gets cancer at age forty. She's just started chemo and wears a baseball cap to cover her thinning hair. She and Betty joke and make us laugh. Carol and Sandra cry a bit. Elana talks about how angry she is. Doris, who is a bingo champion of Southern California, tells us she hasn't had treatment yet because she can't find a doctor she likes and trusts. Polly talks about the changes in her diet, the herbs she's growing, her mother's death from brain cancer a few years ago. Beth talks about the history of cancer in her family, her wonderful boyfriend, her friends helping her out.

In the weeks to come, ten weeks, every Tuesday at six, this room filled with these women will become my refuge; my place to say whatever I need to say and be understood.

What I don't know this first night is that seven of us will stick together after the group sessions end, we'll have potluck dinners at each other's houses and e-mail each other regularly, we'll call ourselves the Bosom Buddies, and in the next five years we'll go through two weddings and one funeral together.

We loved our house, I loved my garden, but these didn't seem enough; now we needed community, like-minded company. We both needed support and a place that would leave us alone to work on what was essential, which was trying to understand what was happening to us, feeling our way, finding how to live well. Who knew how much time we'd have? Nothing, nothing erodes one's patience like that question.

—Mark Doty, *Heaven's Coast*

There is a certain clubbiness to illness that is one of its few saving graces. At the blood bank, all the autologous donors (those giving blood for their own eventual use) have a known problem and a scheduled date for some kind of major procedure. You can talk about your own troubles and listen to other people's, which is no small comfort, since at this stage of things, a couple of weeks or so before surgery, I had pretty well exhausted the number of friends and acquaintances who wanted to hear about my cancer.

—Michael Korda, *Man to Man, Surviving Prostate Cancer*

. . . a kindly lady from Reach for Recovery came to see me . . . "Look at me," she said, opening her trim powder-blue man-tailored jacket and standing before me in a tight blue sweater, a gold embossed locket of no mean dimension provocatively nestling between her two considerable breasts. "Now, can you tell which is which?"

I admitted that I could not. In her tight foundation garment and stiff, uplifting bra, both breasts looked equally unreal to me. But then I've always been a connoisseur of women's breasts, and never overly fond of stiff uplifts. I looked away, thinking, "I wonder if there are any black lesbian feminists in Reach for Recovery?"

I ached to talk to women about the experience I had just been through, and about what might be to come, and how were they doing it and how had they done it. But I needed to talk with women who shared at least some of my major concerns and beliefs and visions, who shared at least some of my language. And this lady, admirable though she might be, did not.

—Audre Lorde, *The Cancer Journals*

In a recent television commercial for a company that makes drugs for cancer, a woman talks about being diagnosed with breast cancer. Looking into the camera, she says she felt as if she had fallen off a boat, leaving everyone else on board, and she didn't know how to swim.

You, or the person you love, hears a diagnosis, has an accident, and yes, it's like falling overboard into very deep, cold water. Meanwhile there goes real life, the boat full of healthy people sailing off into the distance, as you flounder around, cold, terrified of drowning, and very much alone.

Write about what you did when you fell off the boat. Did you call for help? Did you feel as if you were drowning? Or did you figure out how to swim?

Bob writes: *Falling off the boat. That's what she did. Took a dive, didn't ask permission, just went for it. If she had been a child who couldn't swim, parental instinct would have me overboard. No courage required in the rescue . . . Yes, the boat goes on. I'm glad I decided to dive overboard with her. We can spend time stranded on the shore, happy for a beautiful sunset. Hoping for meaning and spiritual peace. Yes, there's a loss, a visible scar, still a bit of—why us, we're still parenting. But God knows best, perhaps that boat was bound to break up on the next rapids.*

Laura writes: *What did I do when I fell off the boat? I picked up the phone and called 75 people or more and told them I had cancer. Being a mother with minor children, cancer didn't just happen to me. I was not free to wallow in grief or cry hysterically or stop and give up. I forced myself to keep going for the sake of my family. I wanted to give my (women mostly) friends an opportunity to help me. It was the best decision. Cancer turned me into a fence with the slats falling down and my friends were the persistent ivy twining up and holding me up. Cancer stopped time like an escalator that doesn't move and my friends reminded me to lift my feet. Cancer took my breath away and my friends blew in my face, and stopped long enough to breathe with me.*

Write about who you pick up the phone to call, or e-mail, or meet for coffee.

Write about your ivy—who holds you up? Write about a community that you feel connected to.

John writes: *I have my community of family and good friends, the ones who still call. These are the people I can call and ask to come visit on chemo day when there is enough of me left and the strength to visit. Only a few people seemed to drop out of my world, scared by the cancer bogeyman. And wonderfully I have added The Wellness Community—especially those people we've met there who have become good friends— friends I enjoy hanging out with.*

Tippy writes: *The support I feel here is the closest I've ever come to a sorority. Once a month I feel like we're wearing pajamas . . . sharing our deepest thoughts.*

Linda, a published poet, who works at The Wellness Community, writes a poem:

If family could be my community
if all the plants in my garden could be my community
I would not have need to join with people
who travel narrow paths of disease and memory,

but that is not the case.
The garden is not enough.
My family is too much dispersed
in geography and disposition,

so I need the writers and musicians.
I need the people who stretch their borders
and their minds into corners
on a zafu or a white page,
people who jump into the jaws of jazz.

I cherish my connection to these people
who examine and struggle alone and with each other
people who are willing to admit that they are afraid
of their fear, people who like to eat food from other countries
and explore the country of their minds.

If you don't have support or community, write about that. How it feels, what being alone is like. Put into words what your ideal community would be, what could make you feel nurtured, understood, and connected.

18

BOMB DRILLS AND SEX

My own true body, the body that makes love, has gone into hibernation. What I have instead is this public body, owned by doctors, examined and touched, x-rayed, carved, and stitched, written about on charts. This body has breasts that feel as foreign and as far away as Russia.

When you're in physical trouble the privacy of your body, the mystery of it, is invaded. The only way to deal with it is to disconnect from your body.

This does not lead to very sexy feelings. Every time there's a new scare—waiting to hear test results, an unidentified bump or twinge, even just being tired, your body goes into war alert. It's like being a little kid in the fifties when there were bomb drills and you had to jump under your desk and cover your head when the alarms went off. Sex is about oblivion, not about being tense and ready to jump under your desk. Your skin is supposed to be pleasureful, not the site of a potential disaster.

Tuesday nights with my Wellness Community group is the only place I feel comfortable discussing any of this. Some of us pull up our sweaters and show each other our scars. Carol cries and says she can no longer get undressed in front of her husband, she feels deformed. Beth's wonderful boyfriend has disappeared.

Then one day I'm taking a shower and R. is watching me. When I get out he says, "You look like a young girl."

Well, I know this is a wee bit of an exaggeration, if not an outright hallucination, but he's serious. And he says it with such sweetness in his voice that finally, at last, after all these weeks, I begin to move out of my frozen body.

I remember a wonderful book I read years ago by Joan and Robert Parker about her breast cancer and the first time they made love. "We'll pretend we're very old people," she told him, "and we'll do the whole thing very gingerly. Very carefully."

So we do it gingerly, very carefully, and very tenderly.

Carefully, gently, thoughtfully, they made love. Part of Joan analyzed and recorded. That's okay. That doesn't hurt. This is all right. By Christ, we're doing okay . . . I wonder if he minds. I wonder if he can tell that one boob is a falsie? Does he feel the difference? Is he fantasizing some zoftig two-boobed lovely? A complete woman? I hope not; I don't blame him but I hope he isn't.

"You okay?" he said.

"Yes," she said.

He's concentrating on what's left. She thought. Not what's gone.

Afterward they were quiet in the dark, lying side by side on their backs, holding hands. Upstairs the boys were asleep. From his place under the drape the dog made his sleeping sounds. They were home. They were in a good place. And they would be there tomorrow.

"What do you think?" she said. "What do you think about the one boob?"

He raised one eyebrow in the dark and sucked his cheeks in and said, "Frankly, my dear, I don't give a damn."

—Joan H. Parker and Robert B. Parker,
Three Weeks in Spring

Donning that condom was a little like wearing an asbestos suit and trying to forget you're walking through fire. Our self-consciousness became a third party who crawled into bed with us, cajoling and cheering and shouting directions, however well intended, it's presence between the sheets was distracting. It took several months after we'd taken our HIV tests for our sex life to return to normal. I realize that many people entertain grave doubts as to the normalcy of same-sex relationships in the first place, and in some sense, it was precisely my internal arguments with such people that helped restore my sex life with Brian.

—Bernard Cooper, *Truth Serum*

I told her, too, about making love: always on my back, unable to kneel, and if I lay on my stomach I could barely move my lower body and had to keep my upper body raised with a suspended push-up. I did not tell her the true sorrow of lovemaking but I am certain that she knew; it made me remember my legs as they once were, and to feel too deeply how crippled I had become.

—Andre Dubus, *Broken Vessels*

Stumbling upon the startling statement in a "Chemotherapy and You" brochure: "It is advisable to wear a condom during intercourse for up to 48 hours after treatment, as chemotherapy drugs may be present in sperm," and at once being taken aback and frightened. For me and for Paula, who I may be unwittingly poisoning. "Nobody told me this," I'm thinking, while hurriedly doing the math. I breathe easier when it computes: It's been at least seventy-two hours since my last dose of chemo. So last night was okay. In more ways than one.

—Curtis Pesmen, "My Cancer Story," *Esquire*, September 2001

In the first chapter of *Wild Mind, Living the Writer's Life*, Natalie Goldberg compares the rules of writing practice to sex: keep your hand moving, be specific, lose control, don't think.

Write about what you concentrate on: what's left or what's gone?

Write about your public body. Write about your private body.

Write about erotic thoughts and experiences before your life changed.

Write about afterward.

Keep your hand moving, keep writing. Don't edit, don't think. Be specific. If it gets too personal, you can always tear up the page when you're finished.

Laura's husband, Bob, veers into sex when writing about food in an earlier exercise: *Are there substitutes that don't distort the waistline? Would yoga to excess be as satisfying? I know strength exercises can release those endorphins of good feeling. Erotic consumption is a wonderful substitute—But that requires more planning, and getting a partner in the mood takes a lot more effort than opening the refrigerator and reaching into the cookies.*

Jean writes: *We met with a nurse who explained the procedure and rules for chemo from the fact that visitors cannot sit on the nurse's rolling stools to dozens of my restrictions . . . Steve asked about having sex. The nurse stuttered. "We usually don't recommend sex during chemotherapy treatment, but you're young and it will be a couple of months." She rushed off to find a brochure from the American Cancer Society about sex during cancer. She told us to ask my oncologist if we had any more questions. I couldn't even imagine—my oncologist seems only a little bit older than my son. I asked Steve to read the brochure. He told me it said it was dangerous to have sex during chemotherapy. We remembered those rules about not having intercourse after having a baby and we improvised.*

19

ON THE BEACH

*Y*ou *know there's a reason the radiation department is in the basement of the* hospital. You know there's a reason that everyone leaves the room and talks to you through an intercom while the machine lowers down like a spaceship, whirs, and zaps you. But you don't want to think about it.

I close my eyes for the seconds I'm being zapped and try to do a very positive visualization. The sun is healing me. I'm on a beach, listening to the surf, feeling tropic breezes against my skin, the sand is warm, the sun is hot. But the fact is I'm in Torrance, California, having killer rays beamed into my flesh, and nobody has a clue what this will result in, twenty years down the road. The point, I guess, is to be around in twenty years to find out.

Then, oddly, the routine of coming here every weekday at three-thirty becomes ordinary. I like the nurses and technicians, my doctor. My breast grows pink in the days and weeks to come, feels a little tender as if I were indeed at the beach every day with only my left breast exposed to the hot sun. I rub special lotion on it. There's no pain, and the dreaded radiation exhaustion never comes. I'm not tired. In fact it's a nonevent.

Written in my appointment book for three-thirty every weekday: radiation.

There's a comforting familiarity to it.

*You go through radiation . . . Then your immune system is all you have
to kill the aberrant cells, which you imagine as sinister and black-clad,
smoking cigarettes as they cluster in the dark S & M club of your body.*
   —Melissa Bank, *The Girls' Guide to Hunting and Fishing*

*Almost all the cancer self-help books talked about visualization: they
claimed some patients were able to help and even cure themselves by
relaxing deeply and imagining the white blood cells of their immune
system battling the cancer cells . . . What was I to imagine? If I hoped
my body was cancer-free, should I be imagining cancer cells within it at
all, even if they were being destroyed by whatever white creatures I
chose as a metaphor for my white blood cells? Or should I just think of
torrents of water pouring through my system and cleansing it? Or music
to bring everything into harmony? Did you have to be able to visualize
your bones, blood, organs and cells accurately or could you sort of fudge
it? And what was the best creature to choose as your inner ally?*
   —Juliet Wittman, *Breast Cancer Journal, A Century of Petals*

*The kind of imagery that is important to me is what is evoked
spontaneously from people. Each person's imagery is unique and has a
life of its own. Even if two people have the same image, like the image of
a wolf, that wolf has a totally different meaning for one person than for
another. As you evoke these images, it's almost as if a movement
towards wholeness is also being evoked. That movement is there in
everybody, sometimes weak and sometimes strong, but it's there. It's like
the will to live.*
   —Rachel Naomi Remen, M.D., *Healing and the Mind*
   (quoted by Bill Moyers)

*I saw the word RELAX as pillows—huge, overstuffed furniture pillows
in the shape of the letters. I would imagine crawling into each letter and
finding a place in the letter where I could curl up and feel safe and
relaxed . . . I would be so happy in that little relaxed pillow, crawling all
around in there. When I got tired of doing that, I turned it into an air
mattress that floated in the pool on a clear, bright, shiny day. I'd lie on*

the word RELAX in the pool and let the sun warm me. Once again I
would feel safe and calm.

—Gilda Radner, *It's Always Something*

When I was going through my divorce a friend gave me a tape that I listened to every night when I woke up at three and couldn't go back to sleep. The tape was of a man's voice telling me to relax my toes, the soles of my feet, my heels, ankles . . . and upward, all the way up to the top of my head. It wasn't a very professional or polished tape, he had a thin, rather strange voice, but he always put me to sleep. God knows what the neighbors thought.

Sometimes in the workshop we do a relaxation exercise before writing as a way to get into the moment, to let go of everything that happened so far today, and the anticipation or worries about what's happening later. We count breaths, five slow counts in, hold for five, and then exhale slowly to the count of five. Then focusing on the toes, soles of the feet, heels, ankles, just like my man on the tape. You picture each part of your body relaxing as you focus on it. When you reach the top of your head, you take more deep counted breaths and imagine inhaling energy, and then exhaling all the tension in your body.

Dave later writes a poem about relaxation:
> *For when I stop,*
> *and hear and feel,*
> *my body will lead me to*
> *the quietest of meditations,*
> *and the world begins,*
> *from deep within my core.*

Relaxation also prepares you for guided imagery—visualizing something that's positive, that can lead to new insights, or simply help you to feel better. One visualization we do is of a special place, real or imaginary. It could be the beach, a favorite room in your house, the mountains, a cottage in the woods, or a place that you make up.

Paying attention to your senses—what you see, hear, smell, touch and taste—try to make this place as safe and beautiful as you can, full of wonderful things to look at, soothing sounds, delicious smells, and objects and fabric that feel good to touch, wonderful things to eat and drink. Create a place so real and rich in detail that you can slip back into it whenever you need to.

Writing down all the details you visualize will make the place more real to you, more accessible, and easier to use as a refuge when you need one. Write what you see when you look around the place. Write what your senses pick up. Is there anyone else there? Write down whatever images come to you.

Margie writes about going to a beautiful mountain, clean air, fresh blue skies, and at the top of the mountain, sitting at a long table filled with delicious food, she finds all the people she has ever loved and lost, having a party, inviting her to join them.

20

ROWING TOWARD THE RAFT

And now finally real life begins to loom larger than being a cancer patient. I haven't missed teaching any of my weekly classes, though the first two weeks after surgery, when my left arm was sore and stiff, Nancy, one of my students, drove me to class. I write every day when I'm not teaching. And then there's radiation every day at three-thirty.

I feel as though I've been rowing toward a raft, trying to reach a safe place, trying to get out of cold, deep water.

R. travels a lot for business and when he's gone I stay in my own house. My office is here, and it's home for Stuart and Charlotte, my cats. I work on my novel and write terrible essays about the urgency of giving yourself monthly exams and not relying solely on mammograms. They're more like strident lectures than essays. All day there's constant pounding as the new roof goes on my house.

Our wedding plans move forward. The Episcopal Church requires prenuptial counseling, no matter what your age or how wise and experienced you consider yourself to be. R. and I love taking the compatibility tests, both of us relieved to learn that after long marriages in which the word *compatible* did not instantly spring to mind, that with the right person, we are indeed compatible. The priest says diplomatically that it's interesting to counsel couples who are a little older than the average bride and groom. Younger couples have so many issues, and we seem to be such good friends. R. and I agree; we're best friends.

When I went through my divorce, I kept a journal on a daily, sometimes hourly, basis. I filled page after page, notebook after notebook, riding a roller coaster of emotion. I became addicted to writing everything down. Last February—once I got the nerve to write the word *cancer* in my journal, I wrote a lot about it. Riding not so much a roller coaster but more of an escalator of emotion. Recently, though, my journal entries are getting briefer, filled more with daily details than great arcs of emotion. I realize that life does indeed (if you're lucky) go on.

I ask myself in my journal: *But what have I learned from all this?* I was very clear on what I learned from the pain of a failed marriage and divorce, but what does having a disease that threatens my life teach me?

That this isn't a dress rehearsal, this is it, real life? Wake up and smell the coffee? Stop and smell the roses? What doesn't kill you makes you stronger?

Am I learning only clichés?

What has this journey been about? Am I reaching a raft, or is this finally the shore of real life?

R. takes me on a weekend trip to Santa Barbara for my birthday. I'm fifty-eight years old. An age most women keep secret, or at least don't announce to the world. But all I can think of on this birthday, turning this age, is that *I'm alive.* I'm paying attention to every perfect, and not so perfect, precious moment.

Maybe what I'm learning is gratitude.

I had witnessed the progress of fatal illnesses so many times that I knew what was coming: When I finally understood that my disease could kill me, I had to go through the process of watching myself die, of seeing my life for what it was, and setting aside my dreams. Only after I had buried myself could I take stock of what was left, put the sadness aside, and go forward. But I could not do this alone.

—Jerri Nielsen, M.D., *Ice Bound: A Doctor's Incredible Battle for Survival at the South Pole*

*Besides, for all the things I've lost, there's so much that's been gained.
My stroke came as a punctuation mark in the course of a busy life. At
the time, I thought it was a full stop, but it turned out to be a comma, or
at worst an exclamation point.*

—Robert McCrum, *My Year Off, Recovering Life After a Stroke*

*This time seems so powerful . . . I see without the burden of time past or
visions of the future. Piles of dirty clothes in a basket assail my eyes with
such color. The bamboo blinds hanging on three windows change with
every outside light, throwing patterns of slants on the bookcase. Painted
sticks of sunshine and dark. My soft orange glass-shaded lamp slips me
so gently into twilight and then darkness. How I love.*

—Sandy Dennis, *A Personal Memoir*

There was a personal essay published in the *Los Angeles Times* last year
entitled "Five Things Cancer Taught Me" by Jennie Nash about getting
breast cancer at age thirty-five. It's a quirky and funny piece, yet also
serious and moving (and turned out to be the start of a book for her).
The five things she learned included realizing that imagined evils are
worse than actual ones, that the Victoria's Secret catalog never stops
coming no matter what you're going through, and that her story is
important to tell. Since good writing always inspires our own writing, I
use this essay in the workshop as an example of writing about illness.

Write five things you've learned from your illness, your injury, or
from the person you love who's hurt or ill.

Deb writes six things she learned:

- *Without hair, I look like a character from Star Trek, The Next
  Generation.*

- *This chemo is making me pee red. Urine really does look best in
  yellow.*

▮ *I don't like living alone.*

▮ *Locked inside this radiation vault, I am safe from an earthquake. You unlucky stiffs in the booth, however, are not.*

▮ *My coworkers in the hip world of advertising are uncomfortable with me now.*

▮ *Soap operas aren't so bad. In fact, I want to borrow one of their tricks where they replace one actor with another to play a certain character. You know, where the voice-over says, "The part of Cassandra, the evil vixen, will now be played by Eve Jones." So as I'm about to enter that chemo room we hear, "The part of Deb, the cancer patient, will now be played by Eve Jones, while Deb goes on with a healthy life."*

Carolyn writes:

1. *I am so lucky: that list of things I scurried to do before I died—I got to do all of them, and I'm still here!*

2. *I got a new word in my vocabulary: "no" followed by no explanation (and then Carolyn gets stuck in the exercise but continues on anyway).*

3. *No thoughts are coming.*

4. *I don't feel like doing this exercise right now.*

5. *The flower we see is only a moment in its life—it's living, breathing, changing life— like mine. Any flower is the culmination of its flower parents that dropped fertile seed which responded to the darkness and moistness of the earth: these moments are the flower. And when it pokes its first leaves through the earth, this is the flower. And when its greenness stretches to the sun and drinks the rain and breathes deeply of my CO_2 when I lean over to admire it, this is the*

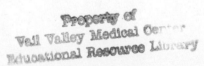

flower. And when the bud blooms into color, thriving in its parent stage, this is the flower. And when it gets old and goes to seed itself and then returns to join the compost heap, this is the flower.

Laura writes:

1. *Negative People Are Very Valuable*

   I told so many friends about my cancer. The "positive-thinkers" were sometimes devastated and unable to help. My grumpy, cranky friends were able to quickly roll up their sleeves and chip in. They expect the worst of life and appreciated the challenge.

2. *I Cannot Control the Future*

   Of course I always knew this, but getting cancer at 44 made the point even more obvious.

3. *I Am Strong and Loved*

   Looking back, I can see what a brave patient I was. Now post-cancer, I am dealing with the messy emotions I postponed while I was being so courageous and positive during treatment. I would be overwhelmed by the outpouring of love from dozens of friends and then suddenly engulfed by the dark fear of death.

4. *I Am Creating Positive Memories for My Children.*

   Not all positive, but powerful memories. I am teaching them to survive, to persist, to do what is possible with the limitations of my fatigue and my sadness.

Maybe you feel you haven't learned a damn thing from whatever it is you're going through. In that case, write five things you haven't learned.

Write five things you wish you never had to know.
Write five things you want to find out.
Or go on to six things or thirty, or write just one.

Dave writes: *Consumed is how I am learning to live, remission or not, real or not, all or not, consumed by this moment. Living as if a high school kid, a whole calendar ahead, a cat with nine lives, a life full of fire, more to come, more to come.*

21

Into the Future: Old Ladies
Wearing Sun Hats, Trailing Scarves

*A*nd *suddenly radiation treatment is over. For the past three months I've* been in the middle of all this drama—surgery, doctors behind every door, urgency, radiation every day. Such busyness and focus, such attention! I don't realize until it's over that there was a certain comfort in treatment. *Something was being done.*

But now, God only knows what's happening in my body. No one is paying attention to it. And of course my days of playing the brave cancer patient are over. Back to real life 24/7.

R. and I want to sell our houses and find one house to live in together. This isn't easy. He likes big houses with views, and I like small cozy houses with privacy. He's also allergic to my cats which is one reason I've kept my own house. In April our Realtor, his sister-in-law, finds a 1929 house in Santa Monica she thinks we'd both like. And she's right, it's got something for each of us—a view and privacy, lots of space but small and cozy rooms. There's even a special floor for my office and Stuart and Charlotte. I fall madly in love with the house even though it clearly needs major restoration.

And then this awful bad-attitude, rude, party-pooper voice pops up in my head and says: *Yeah, but will you be alive when it's finished?*

I call up my cousin Sally, the most positive person on the planet, and tell her about the house, how wonderful it is, but that the future is so uncertain, how can R. and I take on this huge project? What if I have a recurrence? What if I, well you know, like die in the middle of it?

Sally tells me what I want to hear—that of course I'm not going to die while restoring the house. I'll live to grow old in it.

Then we spin a fantasy of being eccentric old ladies walking on the beach in Santa Monica, wearing huge sun hats, trailing scarves, drinking wine as we watch the sun set, being outrageous and raucous, embarrassing our children, laughing a lot, writing and painting and living to be a hundred.

But how do you survive cancer? That's the part no one gives you any advice on. What does it mean? Once you finish your treatment, the doctors say, You're cured, so go off and live. Happy trails. But there is no support system in place to help you to deal with the emotional ramifications of trying to return to the world after being in a battle for your existence.

—Lance Armstrong, *It's Not About the Bike*

Lying awake in the gray hours of the morning, I heard a hissing little voice, insinuating, familiar, from the depths of my own being. And what it was saying, over and over again, was simply, "Metastasis. Metastasis."

Over the next few weeks it returned periodically, like a nightmare, until the day I confronted it. "You're nothing," I told this sinister, deathly presence. "Nothing at all. That's only a word."

—Juliet Wittman, *Breast Cancer Journal, A Century of Petals*

Like a ghost, that party-pooper voice loses definition and power when exposed to the light of paper, or to a computer screen. Or to the ears of a positive friend.

Write out what that negative voice in your head is saying. What's the worst thing it tells you? Talk back to it.

It's like the carping critic in your head when you write. Or a crazy dog. Trying to hide it in the closet and keep it quiet just doesn't work. Let it bark, let it run around the room and chew up some old shoes and act ridiculous. It'll get tired and after a while curl up in the corner and go to sleep.

Audrey writes about hearing voices from her past saying: . . . *should and have to, ought to and must, you're wrong, that's silly, that can't be done, be careful, are you sure that's okay, you're not doing it right, if I were you I would have done thus and so, that would be fine if it were an inch shorter or longer, not enough, too much and on and on. Like a caged bird with clipped wings. Now in present life the bird is free and learning to fly.*

Spin a fantasy. Write an image of yourself in the future; the best-case scenario.
    Write about changes you can make in your life.

Anne writes: *Next week I'll be 75 and so I have been saying "No" more frequently. I decided I would make this workshop so I told my daughter I couldn't baby-sit today. I didn't go to church last Sunday. I usually get dressed first thing so I can go out and retrieve the papers. But I went out in my pajamas and slippers—didn't even put my robe on. I'm not going to do things I don't want to do anymore.*

What are your goals, realistic and otherwise? (Otherwise is as important to write about as realistic.)

Laura writes: *I try to believe this is something I will live beyond. When I am in my 60s and 70s and 80s—when my friends get cancer, I'll be able to say, "Oh, yes, I remember cancer, that was decades ago." People will be so amazed that I survived the primitive chemotherapy like we're amazed that doctors used leeches a century ago.*

Write about who or what you go to for comfort and solace.
    Write about the most positive person you know, and why.
    Write about what you see in your mirror.

Jean writes: *My friends are my mirrors. But now they're fun house mirrors that distort the image. They're remembering me from months ago—when I used to be positive before being drained by too much chemo, too many losses, months of no sun, no bare feet, no shopping, saying no to my kids. No no no no no.*

Deb writes: *I stare at my face in the mirror a lot these days. The lines are deeper now, like cuts. I age. I am puffy under the eyes from too little sleep. But I don't want to correct any of it. I am attracted to all that I am as much as I loathe all that I am. I like the anger in me. That lady at work woke up this sleeping giant in me. When she told me about her relative whose breast cancer had recurred after eight years. Eight years.*

Write about what wakes the sleeping giant in you.

22

FROG JOKES AND GUILT

*O*ur *Wellness Community group sessions are almost over—ten weeks together.* And I've begun to feel guilty; I'm one of the oldest in the group, and am having the easiest time with not only breast cancer but also in my personal life. No mastectomy, no chemotherapy, and my wedding coming up in August. I don't know what to do with this guilt. Ruth suggests that I talk about it in group. But to talk about it would seem to compound it. *Not only am I lucky, but now I'm going to whine about it.*

One evening in group, Dee, who is always hip and funny and gives smart, loving feedback to everyone, and who is now in the middle of her chemotherapy and living alone, breaks down and cries for the first time. "I'm just so tired," she says. My heart aches for her. And my guilt goes up another notch.

Four years later when I tell Dee about the guilty feelings I had in group, she'll respond with this e-mail message: "Some of us got hit by more bullets than others; some of us dodged the bullets. Some of us got blown to bits. But none of us escaped the fear, the what-ifs, the how is this going to turn out, which is the biggest horror of cancer. None of us came back the same."

When I thank her for the message, for taking me off the hook of my own guilt, she e-mails back: "What are Bosom Buddies for if they can't help out a fellow Bosom?"

When the group sessions end, we have a potluck supper at my house in Hermosa Beach.

We drink wine and talk about reasons people get cancer. (Telephone wires! Microwave ovens! Deodorant! Wine!) And for some reason we all find this uproariously funny. We share tofu recipes. We tell dirty jokes. R. drops by to meet the women he's heard so much about. He arrives during the dirty jokes, not the recipes. Everybody flirts with him. He flirts back. Polly tells a truly crude and hilarious joke about a frog. I tell the one dirty joke I know. It's a joke that no one has ever, ever found funny except for me. This group laughs. Of course we laugh at everything; it's one of those evenings when there's nothing that's not funny.

Finally, R.'s allergies to my cats kick in, and he has to leave.

Later he tells me he expected a more somber group of women, women who were dealing with serious issues.

Which of course is exactly what we were doing.

&

I have a theory now that cancer cells hate laughter and jokes and songs and dancing. They want to leave when too much of that is going on. They love gloom and depression and sadness and fear, but joy makes them want to move out.

—Gilda Radner, *It's Always Something*

It was easy enough to hope and love and have faith, but what about laughter? Nothing is less funny than being flat on your back with all the bones in your spine and joints hurting. A systematic program was indicated. A good place to begin, I thought, was with amusing movies . . . It worked. I made the joyous discovery that ten minutes of genuine belly laughter had an anesthetic effect and would give me at least two hours of pain-free sleep. When the pain-killing effect of the laughter wore off, we would switch on the motion-picture projector again, and, not infrequently, it would lead to another pain-free interval.

—Norman Cousins, *Anatomy of an Illness*

Thinking all the time about having MS grew tiresome and intrusive, especially in the large and tragic mode in which I was accustomed to

considering my plight. Months and even years went by without
catastrophe (at least without one attached to MS), and really I was
awfully busy, what with George and children and snakes and students
and poems, and I hadn't the time, let alone the inclination, to devote
myself to being a disease. Too, the richer my life became, the funnier it
seemed, as though there were some connection between largess and
laughter, and so my tragic stance began to waver until, even with the
aid of a brace and a cane, I couldn't hold it for very long at a time.

—Nancy Mairs, "On Being a Cripple," from *Plain Text*

Laughter simply feels good; your body, your mind, your heart,
everything in you is engaged and affected. It's like doors opening
and letting in light and air. In the workshop we laugh a lot; it's like
the dark humor of survivors, the laughter of recognition. There are
tears too sometimes, and both the laughter and the tears, as we
write and read aloud, feel comfortable; we become free and easy
with our own emotions, feel cleansed and emptied out. Joni
Mitchell once wrote in a song that laughing and crying are the same
release.

In your notebook keep track of things that strike you as funny—
cartoons, scenes in movies, jokes, stories, things you overhear. Pay
attention the next time you laugh hard and write how it makes your
body feel.

Deb writes a poem about laughter, called "Mom's Movie":

> *When I am burned out,*
> *turned inside out,*
> *I lay narrow next*
> *to you on the couch*
> *to watch some movie that makes you laugh.*
>
> *Oh, how you laugh.*

Ribs rising sending
vibes into me
waking sawed-off bones,
spilling charged-up air
poured out from where
there is no pain.

And when it stops,
and we are still
I see I am born
from you again.

Write about a place where there is no pain.

Write about waking up sawed-off bones with laughter and light.

Linda writes:

> *You pray for laughter. You pray*
> *for the river of forgetfulness to flow*
> *into your life and offer you a ride.*

Stephen King in *On Writing, A Memoir of the Craft,* addresses the other side of the emotional coin. When he gets up for the first time after his terrible accident, he sits on the commode weeping. "You try to tell yourself that you've been lucky, most incredibly lucky, and usually that works because it's true," he writes. "Sometimes it doesn't work, that's all. Then you cry."

Write about when you cried in the past, and when you cry now.

Dave writes:

> *I am eight years old*
> *since Stage 2 melanoma*

and six years old
since Stage 4 melanoma.

Naps I take,
and I did then too.
Even before
Mrs. Karpel, my kindergarten teacher,
insisted that boys take naps and don't cry.
Well, I have always cried,
and now I nap.

WHO AM I NOW?

As the weeks since my diagnosis turn into months, I am less inclined to broadcast the fact that I've been treated for breast cancer. It's not that I'm keeping it secret, it's just that I'm not so eager to make this an ongoing part of my identity. I even begin to question the label *breast cancer survivor*. Am I tempting fate with that phrase? And then, if I don't survive, if I'm one of those lazy patients who hasn't been able to conquer negative thoughts and get her act together—am I a loser? A breast cancer survivor who ended up failing the ultimate survival test? Got voted off the island?

To give myself this label overshadows who I think I really am—writer and teacher, mother of my girls and about-to-be-wife of R. Somewhere down this list I am a person who *had* breast cancer. I am also someone who had her appendix out, broke a toe, had a hysterectomy, got a divorce. There's a whole list of stuff I'd prefer to leave in the past, not drag into the future with me.

What words do I use for what has happened to me? The words *in remission* scare me; it sounds so temporary, as if cancer is simply lurking in the wings waiting to reappear.

It's like that old joke about Vietnam: we should have just declared ourselves the winner and gotten out.

I am someone who had breast cancer. I won. I'm getting out.

First, the matter of semantics. I am a cripple. I choose this word to name me. I choose from among several possibilities, the most common of which

*are "handicapped" and "disabled." I made the choice a number of
years ago, without thinking, unaware of my motives for doing so. Even
now, I'm not sure what those motives are, but I recognize that they are
complex and not entirely flattering. People—crippled or not—wince
at the word "cripple," as they do not at "handicapped" or "disabled."
Perhaps I want them to wince. I want them to see me as a tough
customer, one to whom the fates/gods/viruses have not been kind, but
who can face the brutal truth of her existence squarely. As a cripple, I
swagger.*

—Nancy Mairs, "On Being a Cripple," from *Plain Text*

*Have one good cry, if the tears will come. Then stanch the grief, by
whatever legal means. Next find your way to be somebody else, the next
viable you—a stripped-down whole other clear-eyed person, realistic as
a sawed-off shotgun and thankful for air, not to speak of the human
kindness you'll meet if you get normal luck.*

—Reynolds Price, *A Whole New Life*

*Poets work at making language new by making it vivid and dramatic;
I approached the task of making the self new by making it vivid and
dramatic with as much dedication as any fledgling poet. If I wanted
women to like me, I thought, then I had to confront myself—both as I
was, standing on those double long-legged braces with crutches thrust
beneath my shoulders, and as I wanted to be, a man able to define
both limitation and possibility for himself. How could I exploit the
physical powers I had lost? Like Lermontov, I needed to create a hero
for our time. Only in my case, the hero had to be me.*

—Leonard Kriegel, *Flying Solo*

Someone once asked Picasso how he managed to be so creative and
inventive in his old age, and he said, "It takes a long time to become
young."

Remember when you were a little kid and writing and painting were something to do for fun? Kids don't think writing poetry is a big deal, it's a game.

Think of this as another game. You can be as silly or as weird or as serious as you wish.

You start the first line with the words: *I used to be—*

Start the next line with: *But now I am—*

Try writing ten lines alternating between what you used to be and what you are now. See if you can come up with a different image each time.

You can be more literal with this (*I used to be a fairy princess*, writes Nancy, *but now I am a mortal.*) or you can get into metaphor and go from being a fountain pen to a swimming pool, or from a carrot to a waltz. You don't have to try to explain it with logic. Whatever image pops into your mind, trust it. Have fun with it.

My heart was once captured forever by a second grader who wrote: *I used to be a vegetarian/But now I'm a rabbit's foot.*

Bob writes:

I used to be a weird child prodigy, but I gave it up in a desperate search for acceptance.

I used to be shy and self-conscious, but now I inflict myself on everyone I meet.

I used to be a great lover, but now I have three children, four computers, two TV's and a VCR.

I used to be rich and affluent, but now I pay for ballet lessons and private college.

I used to be sarcastic, but now I'm just a seeker of irony.

Valerie writes her own version of this exercise:

I used to be fairly confident of the goodness of life. Now, I am more so. Why?

I used to be shy. Now I seek out human contact constantly. Why?

I used to be unable to envision my own demise. I still can't. Why?

I used to think there was time enough for everything. Now I know there isn't but I still don't get a lot done. Why?

I used to find it easy to imagine comfort peace and rest. Now I can't. Why?

I used to be afraid of death. Now I'm more afraid of the dying. And I know why.

Carolyn e-mails me copies of her writing from the last workshop. "If you ever are inclined to repeat these words," she says in a note, "please BE SURE TO DELETE MY NAME or to use a pseudonym. I am not out of the cancer closet, as it were, and my diagnosis is still very private to me."

In response to the writing exercise question: What words do I use to describe having cancer? she wrote: *I had cancer. I keep having it, apparently. I used to have had it once; that was hard, but OK. I didn't want to be known as a victim OR a survivor—It was life changing and generated the person I wanted to become. I wasn't a "survivor"; I was becoming Myself. Then the second diagnosis: POOF! All prior meanings vanished, popped like a bubble. Now what is cancer; is it an identity? I'm trying to be finished, this being a cancer patient. I thought I was in remission. I liked that identity A LOT. Is it like trying to stop smoking, where you "stop" 12 different times in your life and so "stop" starts having this weirdly different meaning. How can I be in remission, "again"? My choices of words are very few so far.*

What words do you use for your illness or injury?

In answer to this question, Nancy writes another poem, again entitled "Diagnosed":

DIAGNOSED; to recognize (as a disease) by signs and symptoms.
Webster's Ninth New Collegiate Dictionary
There, now we all know the definition.
It sounds so clinical, so distant.
To be diagnosed,
recognize—something has been discovered,
but keeping "it" away from me.
I've only been diagnosed. I'm still safe. I have a diagnosis.
The words choke me as I say them.
Fear grips my guts.

Eight months later I can actually say "I have lymphoma."
I do not embrace it.
The words make me squirm beneath their weight.
I have a disease and it happens to be cancer.

A small step that has taken Herculean effort.
I've stopped fighting the diagnosis. I now fight the disease.

Write about surviving. Do you put it in the present or in the past tense?

Laura writes: *Now should I say survived cancer (past tense) or survives cancer (present tense)? I like the present tense better. It is what I am doing right now—they don't speak of cures much in "my" type of cancer anyway. I am the mother who survives cancer to transform into the grandmother who tells stories and survives cancer to mutate further into the great-grandmother who creates memories and survives cancer.*

A Spanish-speaking woman, Clara, writes only in English in the workshop. She tells me it keeps the cancer at a distance. It's not in her own language. She puts all the words of cancer into another language, English.

"English is not close to my heart," she says.

24

Blue Fingers and Brave Buddies

An early-June afternoon, two months before the wedding, and I'm driving around doing errands. Life is good, and I'm grateful. R. and I have just returned from a long Memorial Day weekend in Colorado. The wedding invitations are at the printer, I've hired a caterer for the dinner at R.'s house after the church ceremony and arranged for the music. We're about to close the deal on the house in Santa Monica. I'm teaching a weekend seminar soon. Tonight I'm going out to dinner with the Bosom Buddies.

Last weekend in Colorado, R. and I arranged to have my wedding ring, a plain silver band, made by a silversmith in Ouray. As I think about this, happy about the ring—I like knowing the name of the person who's making my wedding ring and the fact that my mother's silver ring is being melted down and added to it—I glance at my left hand on the steering wheel and notice it's puffy. Ominously puffy. It looks like a pincushion without the pins. All the bones and veins in my left hand have suddenly disappeared.

I know instantly what's happened; as if I knew this would happen, not just feared it, but somehow knew. As if I'd been waiting for it. The true antidote for guilt. The other shoe dropping. Dropping on a bright June afternoon two months before my wedding.

I head home to call my doctor for an immediate appointment.

What I think it is, what I know it is, is lymphodema—a disfiguring swelling that comes from lymph fluid not being able to drain properly. I've read long lists of warnings for breast cancer patients to avoid the possibility of it suddenly appearing. You can get it immediately after surgery or radiation, or even years later. To avoid it, you're not to carry anything heavy on the side you had surgery, nor have blood pressure taken on that side, no IVs, no tight rings, always wear gloves gardening, beware of high altitudes and sun, take care of burns and scratches that could become infected. In other words, your arm should be placed in bubble wrap for the rest of your life.

Did I carry something heavy with my left arm? Did I ignore a scratch or burn? The trip to Colorado—we spent time in the sun, we were at ninety-five hundred feet. Did the altitude trigger it? With soap, I take off the tight ring on the forefinger of my left hand.

My surgeon tells me to come right in. And when he looks at my puffy hand—the hand whose veins I used to hate, a work hand, a plain hand, a bony hand, that now I would give anything to get back, he says, yes, it looks like lymphodema and gives me the name of a physical therapist who deals with this at a nearby treatment center. Meanwhile, he tapes my hand and wrist.

I realize that everyone has a specialty, and those who might be artists when it comes to carving cancer out of your breast might not have a grip on taping your hand for lymphodema. By the time I go out to dinner with the Bosom Buddies the tips of my fingers have turned blue.

All of us in the group share a crazed fear of side effects, of feeling vulnerable again, of not having cancer over and done with. And they understand the seriousness of getting lymphodema. They also understand that it can't be good thing to have blue fingers, so they loosen the bandages for me.

Though sinking into abject self-pity over this new development (how will R. put the silver wedding band on my sausage finger?), I also realize how lucky I am to have these women in my life. These are the women who teach me courage. These women who understand how I feel, who will stick with me no matter how deep I sink into feeling sorry for myself about this, who listen and don't offer glib words to make themselves comfortable.

I think I have no real escape except through this. These few fragile words I can manage every day. I must think, I must let myself explore what I'm feeling and thinking. I need to explore that black territory. . . .
—Sandy Dennis, A Personal Memoir

I have forced myself to begin writing when I've been utterly exhausted, when I've felt my soul as thin as a playing card . . . and somehow the activity of writing changes everything.
—Joyce Carol Oates, quoted in Writing Changes Everything

It may prove impossible because my head feels so queer and the smallest effort, mental or physical, exhausts, but I feel so deprived of my self being unable to write, cut off since early January from all that I mean about my life, that I think I must try to write a few lines every day.
—May Sarton, After the Stroke

"You were the most beautiful woman in the room that night, Jennie, and the most courageous. A lot of women in your shoes wouldn't have even shown up, let alone worn that dress."

Courageous? I thought. Courageous? So that was what courage felt like—that rush of judgement to know just what to do—or wear—that sense of satisfaction that nothing—not even cancer—was going to stand in my way of feeling utterly confident, the sweet perfume of feeling completely and totally alive. If that was courage, it suited me as well as the red dress.
—Jennie Nash, The Victoria's Secret Catalog Never Stops Coming

Sometimes it's harder to muster courage for what comes after—awful side effects, difficult treatments—than the diagnosis of the illness or accident itself. Our souls can become thin when pain doesn't end, treatments have side effects, or with the onslaught of more bad news.

Write about the weight of your soul. Write about your soul feeling thin, or fragile, or heavy.

Write about a moment when it seemed everything was under control, but then fell apart again.

Write about something that recently pushed you to the edge.

Write about something you're tired of.

Dave writes:

I am tired of walking through life the wrong way.

I am tired of holding back and not hearing what others live between the lines of their life.

I am tired of disengaging from what is real.

I am tired from not stopping and not resting.

I am tired from not seeing things through.

I am tired of my fog, your fog, and our fog.

Jean writes: *As my sister points out to me, rejecting my fatigue is a way of rejecting my body. I want to learn how to embrace my fatigue, to nurture my fatigue, to accept my fatigue, to wrap my arms around this body that does so much less than I want it to. So much less than I used to insist that it do. To somehow love this body that betrayed me by allowing cancer to grow, to attack, to devastate, to destroy. And now is the time to listen to this body's need to rest.*

If you could manage only a few fragile words every day, what would they be?

Laura writes: *I am here.*

In another writing session she continues: *I am here. I am the mother who tells stories. I am the mother who tells stories and creates memories for her children. I am the mother who tells stories, creates memories for her children and survives cancer. I am the mother who wants far more than a few fragile words. I am greedy and ravenous and excessive. Moderation is not my medium of expression.*

Most of us don't go around thinking about how courageous we are, let alone writing about it. But anyone going through a physical ordeal has moments, if not days, months, years of showing courage. Write about a time when you acted with courage.

Bob writes: *I know it's an ongoing decision to follow her through cancer, and courage comes into play. I've had friends who disengaged from their wives after treatment. Guys who want so much for life to go on as before that acceptance never happens. The outcome of their struggle was sad and missed opportunity for growth. Much of my struggle comes from fighting for the best outcome. How much do I compromise my career, my desire for adventure, travel, excitement? God guides me—but I struggle often with choices.*

John writes: *When I think of courage I think of my dad. He fought and survived Pearl Harbor, Midway, Guadalcanal, and other battles in the Pacific. Until a few years ago I never thought of my dad as my hero or as a particularly courageous man. Fortunately for me, my view has changed and grown. And I am pleased with myself when I think I have handled myself in a difficult time as he would have.*

Tippy writes: *About a month after George died, I went to a screening at the Directors Guild. Chicken Run was playing. I needed a laugh. But I bawled when I saw a man in a wheelchair. I felt I should explain my tears to a woman with whom I struck up an acquaintance. She said that I was so brave. "Huh? Brave?" She said I was brave because she had a friend who hadn't left the house in a year. I suppose it's easy to be courageous when you don't know you are doing so.*

25

FALLING OFF HORSES

*N*ow *I'm afraid I'll look like elephant lady at the altar.*

"I've got to have my arm and hand back to normal in eight weeks," I tell the physical therapist. "I'm getting married."

She measures my hand, my wrist, and various points of my arm, then compares the results to my right side. The numbers aren't good. She's realistic and up front, no sugarcoating about this. Lymphodema can more than triple the size of your arm, she tells me. With treatment I may or may not get the current swelling down, and if I do, I'll always have to take special precautions; when I fly, I'll have to wear a special sleeve and glove. This is a chronic disease and may or may not come back no matter what I do.

In the meantime my hand and arm will be bandaged, I'll have special massages, special exercises. She shows me the way to tape my hand and fingers—across my hand, around each finger, over the top again. It will take me days to learn how to do this properly. The good news is that your fingers don't turn blue when it's done right.

I hate the language of this disease: lymph fluid, drainage massage, compression garments, milk arm. I hate the ugliness of my arm and hand. Though lymphodema won't kill me, in a weird way I'm having a harder time with this than I did with breast cancer. There's no life or death urgency, no drama, just a constant dull ache and this hideous-looking hand and arm. I need role models for how to handle this. Supreme Court justices and movie stars get breast cancer, first ladies, famous novelists, and rock stars, but no one gets lymphodema. Or admits to having it anyway. To my knowledge no one runs or walks or gives galas to raise money for this disease. And lymphodema is not a valid reason to sit around the house reading and smoking pot.

Also it's not terribly sexy to sleep with your heavily bandaged arm propped up on multiple pillows. I feel grotesque and don't want to be touched. R. and I are getting on each other's nerves. "What is it you want from me?" he finally asks.

"The problem is—" I say, and then start to cry. "The problem is you're a guy."

"What the hell do you want me to be?"

"I want you to be a guy, but I want you to act like a woman, to be more sensitive. I want you to know how awful this is."

"I can imagine."

"No you can't. You're a guy."

Things are not helped by the fact that his whole house is being painted inside and out by four polite but very driven Czechoslovakians. The house goes on the market right after the wedding, and everything in it is being packed up in boxes so that the closets, cupboards, and built-in drawers can also be painted. The clothes and books I keep at R.'s house I stuff into my Honda hatchback and return to my own house. I go between our two houses now with tote bags filled with my belongings, but never remembering what I need. My whole life, inside and out, feels as if it's been plunged into chaos. There's no order to it.

Strangers ask me what happened when they see my bandaged hand and arm. I tell them I fell off a horse.

I found myself easily knocked off balance, often by small things that would never have bothered me before. I was acutely sensitive to slights by others. . . . I complained too much. I knew that, but I couldn't seem to stop myself. In Tom's silences, I imagined rebukes. I kept hearing his voice saying: pull yourself together, stop malingering, stop feeling sorry

for yourself. This has gone on long enough. I could only agree. I, too, was sick and tired of being sick and tired.
— Musa Mayer, *Examining Myself: One Woman's Story of Breast Cancer Treatment and Recovery*

For anyone who is for any reason feeling weak in the head it is not advisable to suggest solving a problem that requires choices. Yesterday I spent an hour choosing finally a flowering plum tree, from Wayside Gardens, a birthday gift . . . and two white azaleas. It sounds pleasurable but was actually the hardest hour I have spent for a long time and I cried at the end.
— May Sarton, *After the Stroke*

But I'm sitting here at dinner and failing already, unable to rise above my inner turmoil, hating myself for failing, yet convinced that it's David who views this as a failure. He's a character in my drama without having auditioned for the part. I want to scream at him, Why did you bring me here and why do you expect me to act normal? but I know that these are crazy thoughts, that this dinner plan was mine, as is the expectation that I act in a normal manner. Instead, I play out my inner battle: "I'm sorry I'm being so impossible. Maybe we should leave." "Fine," he replies. I say, "You want to leave because you're furious at me for being such a mess." And on it goes.
— Kathlyn Conway, *Ordinary Life, A Memoir of Illness*

Writing gives order to the great mess of life. This is why writers write. This is why we love to read fiction; there's plot, cause and effect, the inevitability of character and circumstance, things happen for a reason. On the other hand, real life, our life, usually ambles from one thing to another, and it's up to us to make sense of it, and give it meaning.

A terrible accident or illness is chaos, the biggest mess of all. Your sense of order and the predictability of your life is shattered. Cause and effect become more dicey than ever. Writing can help organize chaos and conflicting feelings, can give you some sense of control and meaning. Writing down the details of an experience can sometimes reveal the shape and meaning of what you've been through, and give it clarity.

Think of taking a path through a recent experience you had, as if you'd been on a journey, encountering obstacles. Just a short journey with emotional hurdles—maybe going to a doctor's appointment or to treatment, maybe visiting with a friend or a family get-together. Write about what you needed or wanted. What you were looking for. What was in the way. How you felt.

Nancy writes about her mix of emotions at her father's eightieth birthday:

The family has gathered from near and far. Friends, brothers, cousins, children right down to a few great grands. Under the expansive maples, the tables are cluttered with remnants of the feast . . . Dad is 80. His presents are rolled in a wheelbarrow filled with things he'll use, rakes and shovels, hammers, hoses, work gloves and a Rubbermaid trash can. No clothes for this man, he's worn the same green gardening pants for years. He is a child of the Depression. 'Thou shalt not waste.'

My chest swells with pride for the man who loves to make things grow. His best crop; 7 children. I am proud to be his first. Nancy with the laughing eyes.

Happiness and best wishes, but deep within my chest a poker burns. I look at the father who spawned me and I am envious. I fight tears. The green head of jealousy grows within me. I am ashamed. So I stand under the maples, an arm around a sister's shoulder and tears upon my cheeks. Happiness for him. For me . . . ?

The books say 75% live ten years.

How selfish I am, I tell myself. Time moves slowly as I look around to see the yard with its fruit trees and garden, and the abundant family. Can you feel love and envy at the same time? Happy and sad. Hopeful and anxious. Ashamed and proud. Are my emotions as flawed as my body?

I smile as the tears run down my face. Happy Birthday, Dad. I love you beyond words. The sun breaks through the maples as I wish you many, many more.

In one of my favorite poems, "The Summer Day," Mary Oliver writes about watching a grasshopper; not knowing exactly what prayer is, but that she does know how to pay attention. She ends the poem with these lines:

> *. . . Doesn't everything die at last, and too soon?*
> *Tell me, what is it you plan to do*
> *with your one wild and precious life?*

Write about paying attention. Write about choices. Write about what you plan to do with your one wild, precious life.

Dave writes:

> *Choosing either*
> *Here or there*
>
> *Choosing what I bring*
> *to there or here*
>
> *Choosing better,*
> *Growing wiser.*
> *Choosing.*

Laura writes: *I wanted to live happily ever after. But instead I will struggle and claw, scratch and resist. Fight against the should's—leave my life bare enough so the wants and needs are more obvious. Another decade to help my baby birds learn to fly and then my chance to soar. To choose each day to live an expanded life of whatever I choose. I create my life today and I am creating my future. It may not seem "precious" to you or "wild" to most people. My life is full of breaths, laughter, tears, pushing, taking, feeling, lifting, falling down and getting back up.*

26

Going Crazy on
Hawthorne Boulevard

Twice a week now I have treatment for lymphodema—a drainage massage, which sounds like an awful plumbing procedure, but is in fact quite pleasant; nothing you can see actually drains. The physical therapist also teaches me exercises for my arm using long rubber tubing tied to the doorknob, which, if it comes loose from the knob, boomerangs back at me in a rather alarming way. I'm measured for a compression sleeve, and for a special glove that for some reason is only made (for a shocking price) in Germany and has to be special ordered. In the future I'll wear the compression glove and sleeve whenever I fly, and my recurring nightmare will be that I'm at the airport, about to get on a plane, but I've forgotten the sleeve and glove.

Meanwhile, I wear the bandages wrapped all the way up to my armpit. I vary my routine with curious strangers; sometimes I tell them it was a skydiving accident, sometimes it happened when I was surfing. I've become the Walter Mitty of risky sports.

Gradually the swelling comes down. When I don't wear the bandages I hold my hand out to R. and ask him over and over, does it look swollen? Can you see any swelling? He tells me no, he doesn't, and it's going to be okay. Sometimes at night I ask him if he can feel any lumps in my breasts.

I have my six-month tests, including a mammogram, and on the way to the doctor's office to hear the results I can't breathe. I call one of my daughters on my cell phone. "I'm driving down Hawthorne Boulevard, and I'm going crazy," I tell her.

"Oh, Mom," she says. "It must be scary."

And we talk, and I start to breathe again.

As I wait to see the doctor, every depressing fact I've ever read about breast cancer suddenly rises up amplified by loudspeakers in my head. The five years after cancer treatment with no recurrence and you're home free rule doesn't hold true for breast cancer. Apparently any loose cancer cells from your breast can just sail around in your blood for years, ambush you down the road, show up anywhere, at any time. I've started to read the obituaries in the paper, always checking out any women who have died in late middle age or younger. My worst fears are always confirmed; it's an epidemic.

I've read quotes from a doctor who believes that you can't recover from breast cancer; it'll get you sooner or later. Like a prayer, I repeat the names of very old women I know who had breast cancer and now are surviving into their late eighties and nineties.

Can people just suffocate from fear? Choke on it? Is there a Heimlich maneuver for fear? I'm sure the nurses are smiling at me, being kind and friendly, because they're privy to some dreadful news about the results of my tests. *They know.* It's beyond scary. You heard it once, you can hear it again.

But then, suddenly everything is okay. I go within the space of seconds from tragic possibilities to the deliciousness of ordinary life. Everyone is smiling for real. The mammogram, manual breast check, tumor marker tests—all are negative.

I tell my doctor I've changed my mind about tamoxifen; I want to start taking it.

On the phone my friend expresses relief—now that's over and we can get back to normal. Not so fast. You mean you feel more vulnerable? she asks. I am more vulnerable, I say. This sums it up. Only the women who have breast cancer don't have this attitude of everything's okay now. It will never be quite okay again. Not to dwell on constantly, but each mammogram and the long-delayed report of results brings fear, each pain forecasts some dire efflorescence. Just after treatment, I begin having a

pain in my back, left lung. X-ray reveals nothing. Inside the breast itself, intermittent twinges and pressures, the reassemblage of cells and nerve endings? . . . Each bodily awareness takes its character from cancer— the one that was caught and the one that's running, dodging discovery.

—Carol Simmons Oles, "Lateral Time," from *Living on the Margins, Women Writers on Breast Cancer*

Sometimes fear stalks me like another malignancy, sapping energy and power and attention from my work. A cold becomes sinister; a cough, lung cancer; a bruise, leukemia. Those fears are most powerful when they are not given voice, and close upon their heels comes the fury that I cannot shake them. I am learning to live beyond fear by living through it, and in the process learning to turn fury at my own limitations into some more creative energy. I realize that if I wait until I am no longer afraid to act, write, speak, be, I'll be sending messages on a ouija board, cryptic complaints from the other side. When I dare to be powerful, to use my strength in the service of my vision, then it becomes less important whether or not I am unafraid.

—Audre Lorde, *The Cancer Journals*

Each day is a little longer and lighter, but there are setbacks: a night I cannot sleep; or a new pain in a new place, bringing back the fear of imminent death: I live at the point of anxiety, familiar enough, when a toe cramp fosters speculation about toe cancer. Every day is a seesaw of hope and despair. When I am sore and tired discouragement settles over me like smog over Los Angeles. I suppose I will get better; but then I will be sick again, then die.

—Donald Hall, *Life Work*

Michael J. Fox, in a magazine interview, discussed the book he's writing on his experiences with Parkinson's disease. "I'm writing this book because I have to," he said, "describing things that had only existed as feelings—breaking them down into words, decoding."

Decoding feelings into words; that's what anyone does who picks up a pen to write in a journal about his pain, or sits down at a computer to type out her fear.

Ask yourself questions as you write. What does fear do to my voice, the tips of my fingers? What does despair sound like? What does loneliness taste like? What color is anger? How do I breathe through grief?

What tears you apart?

Susan writes: *I'm afraid of fear. Fear is not going to make me well, but I am afraid at my core. I'm the dog biting its tail. How do I get out? To not to be afraid requires constant vigilance. It's behind every door, every belly laugh, every sunset, every kiss from my lover. It is a black coat. I'm hiding my mortality. Anger would be a blessing—it would cut through my fear.*

Dave writes:

> *I am torn between stopping and thinking right now.*
> *I am torn about going to my center and looking there,*
> *for it is a long commute,*
> *and who knows what is there.*
>
> *I am torn between*
> *accepting all the good news,*
> *and fearing the next exam.*
>
> *I am torn between believing all the good I see,*
> *and knowing free fall loss.*
>
> *I am torn between going where I know*
> *life was, is, and will be good,*
> *rather than staying here,*
> *and not being there.*

For there is bliss,
but I stay amiss, a mess,
and shadow box with life.

Try writing about a specific moment when you felt a strong, painful emotion—anger or fear or grief or any emotion that feels powerful. Write about what triggers it. How your body feels. How your perceptions change. Your senses. Write about how you hide the emotion, or how you let it out.

Deb writes: *I am ripping and scratching at the walls around here, around me. But I don't seem to make much progress at chipping away at the paint, much less the timber. I fight imaginary foes in my garage. In my house. At the playground. At my office. I kick at the air in a roundhouse move I learned in kick boxing. I kick at the darkness. I kick at those walls. I kick until I lose my balance and my breath. I kick until I lose my faith that enemies can even be fought and beaten.*

Write about kicking the darkness.

27

FLAUNTING WHAT'S LEFT

*T*he *lovely, crazy problems of life take over; the breathlessness of the dark* abyss fades like a bad, out-of-control dream.

I focus on wedding details. I deal with the daughter who suddenly announces she doesn't want to be a bridesmaid, a role she considers to be a human altar decoration. I tell her she is not going to be a bridesmaid, simply my daughter standing next to me at the altar.

Nicki, who was maid of honor in my first wedding, wants to have the same role in this wedding. I tell her I'm not having a maid of honor; just our kids standing up with us. She suggests then that she and my cousin Sally be flower girls; mature flower girls. Flower ladies.

There's a UPS strike, and I start to worry if my silver wedding ring will arrive from Colorado.

The Czechoslovakians are finally winding up painting R.'s house, but the kitchen is still packed and useless for cooking. Since there are now some empty rooms in the house, I call Dial-a-Mattress for extra beds for our out-of-town family so they won't have to pay for hotel rooms. The guy who delivers the beds is puzzled by the chaos of the house, the stacks of moving boxes, the empty guest rooms, my bandaged arm. "You moving in or out?" he asks.

"It's a wedding," I say.

Sally arrives from the East Coast. Sunny and Susan give me a bridal shower—the first of any kind of shower I've ever had in my whole life.

My arm and hand have miraculously returned to normal, but I

keep the bandages on to be sure. Tamoxifen is giving me hot flashes, and I fan myself with whatever's at hand to cool off.

My wedding dress is almost finished, sleeveless and simple, kind of a long T-shirt made of cream silk. Diana, who's making it, had breast cancer last year, and like me, was lucky. A lumpectomy, no chemo, then radiation. Besides designing clothes, she volunteers now at the UCLA Medical Center shop for cancer patients that sells prostheses, including fake nipples. When I try on the dress, my nipples stick out, and I ask her, "Do you think I should wear a bra?"

She replies, "Hey, if you've got 'em, flaunt 'em."

I wrote to find beauty and purpose, to know that love is possible and lasting and real, to see day lilies and swimming pools, loyalty and devotion, even though my eyes were closed and all that surrounded me was a darkened room. I wrote because that was who I was at the core, and if I was too damaged to walk around the block, I was lucky all the same. Once I got to my desk, once I started writing, I still believed anything was possible.
—Alice Hoffman, "Sustained by Fiction While Facing Life's Facts," *New York Times* 8/14/00

Writing, in a way, to save my life, to catch what could be saved of Wally's life, to make form and struggle toward a shape, to make a story of us that can be both kept and given away. The story's my truest possession and I burnish and hammer it and wrestle it to make it whole. In return it offers me back to myself, it holds what I cannot, its embrace and memory larger than mine, more permanent . . . Always, always we were becoming a story. But I didn't understand that fusing my life to the narrative, giving myself to the story's life, would be what would allow me to live.
—Mark Doty, *Heaven's Coast*

I write six days a week, long days that often run till bedtime; and the books are different from what came before in more ways than age. I sleep long nights with few hard dreams, and now I've outlived both my parents. Even my handwriting looks very little like the script of the man I was in June of '84. Cranky as it is, it's taller, more legible, with more air and stride. It comes down the arm of a grateful man.

　　　　　　　　　　—Reynolds Price, *A Whole New Life*

I created a story that now exists apart from me. It is a story with which I can live. However devastating or overwhelming the experience was, however unflattering I may sometimes have been as a character, the story is manageable. It is confined within the pages of this book, within the contours of the memories I have captured, within the limits of my ability to understand. This is the story I will carry with me.

　　　　　　—Kathlyn Conway, *Ordinary Life, Memoir of an Illness*

Writing about my illness has provided for me a sort of armature upon which I can deposit, as a sculptor does bits of wet clay, the raw substance of memory and experience to form a new image, a new sense of who I am.

　　　—Musa Mayer, *Examining Myself: One Woman's Story of Breast Cancer Treatment and Recovery*

It's one thing to write in a workshop with everyone reading his or her work aloud and inspiring each other, with energy and camaraderie bouncing off the walls. But what about when you're alone? How do you get inspired to write all by yourself?

Well first of all you don't need to be inspired. Inspiration, a burning need to put pen to paper, or to crank up the computer and pour out ideas and feelings, is not necessary for writing. In fact I can't think of any writers I know who feel a burning need or inspiration to write with any regularity. Maybe in the beginning, when you get a great idea for a book or a story and you have this vision of perfection and feel unusually secure and optimistic about your writing. But perfection, as well as feeling secure and optimistic about your writing, tends to melt under the hard reality of putting words down on the page. Ellen Gilchrist finds it helpful to think of writing in the same terms as building a house: "I like to go out and watch real building projects and study the faces of the carpenters and masons as they add board after board and brick after brick," she writes in *Falling Through Space*. "It reminds me of how hard it is to do anything really worth doing."

Writing can be hard, and the only way around that fact is to write so fast that you get lost in what you're writing. Sometimes inspiration comes as you write. Sometimes not. It doesn't matter. Just think of writing as a practice or a habit. Something you do every day. Dancers go to class every day, musicians practice scales, athletes exercise, actors rehearse. Why do most of us believe that writers should be able to discover the words the first time around?

Finding the right place and a specific time to write can make it easier to get started. Have pens and a notebook, or the computer ready, so that you can slip into your inner world without having to worry about the details of equipment (and possibly giving yourself an excuse not to write: No pens! No paper! How can I write?) The more you write, the more you will write.

If you're a morning person, try writing as early as you possibly can. The minute you wake up is a good time because that carping critic in your head will be half-asleep and too tired to tell you that this is a waste of time, and God, what if someone ever reads this stuff, etc. If you're a night person, try writing when you're tired, just before you go to sleep. Your critic will be too tired to comment. Fool around with different times, see what works best for you.

Write yourself a plan—where and when you're going to write, and for how long. We tend to take the goals we've written down more seriously than the fantasies in our heads.

You don't need major creative moments in order to write. You're just practicing writing. It's not a big deal. Habit, not inspiration, is what's necessary.

The fact is that if you don't make a habit of writing, and write your story it will not get written. It's that simple. If you don't write down the details of your life—the rooms and meals and laughter and gatherings of family and friends, the sunsets, tears, and flashes of understanding—none of it will ever be put down into words and shaped into meaning through language.

Why write?

In her beautiful memoir *Paula*, Isabel Allende writes to her daughter, who is in a coma, "I think that perhaps if I give form to this devastation I shall be able to help you, and myself, and that the meticulous exercise of writing can be our salvation."

In the workshop Deb writes: *Writing is an invitation to visit that internal dark place we might be denying or hiding from. The place where fear and healing live as roommates pissed off at one another. To go there brings peace.*

Dave writes: *Writing joins. Writing includes. When I write, it's for words, words gathered together, sequenced and emphasized . . . Being here, being present, being joined in the moment of a word, in the neighborhood of a sentence, in the community of a paragraph, in a nation of a story, in the world of a book. Writing joins me.*

Carlie writes: *Writing stretches the edges of my cocoon.*

Words connect us, offer us a path out of our cocoons, our isolation, and can become our salvation.

28

TILL DEATH DO US PART

In the same chapel where I sent up prayers for courage exactly six months ago, I now walk down the aisle on my brother's arm, toward R., waiting for me at the altar with our five children standing on either side of him. The pews are filled with our extended family and close friends. The chapel is lit with candles and filled with white flowers. The organist plays "Sheep May Safely Graze." The ring arrived, my dress was finished in time. All around me are the faces of people I love.

The marriage vows from *The Book of Common Prayer* take on a whole new meaning as R. and I repeat them to one another.

Vowing to have and to hold from this day forward till death do us part not only turned out to be inaccurate in my first marriage, but it was also a vow that sounded a lot different when I was twenty-four years old. Death was an event so far off in the future that the whole idea of it was shrouded in mists of time.

But now it's for real. This is the future. And R. is the man who never blinked when he learned I had breast cancer, who would take me with or without breasts, with or without hair and eyebrows, and with an arm and hand that could look like a living pincushion at any instant. This is the man who is vowing to love me, comfort me, honor and keep me, in sickness and in health and forsaking all others, to be faithful to me as long as we both shall live. Until we are parted by death.

This is my one precious life. This is the happy ending to the past six months.

Why me, why am I so lucky? Is it the roll of the big dice in the sky? Genes?

I know how precarious good luck and happiness can be, how fragile. But for this moment in my life, in this celebration of love and commitment and family, there's only joy.

The priest prays: *Grant their wills may be so knit together in your will and their spirits in your Spirit, that they may grow in love and peace with you and one another all the days of their life. Amen*

Maybe faith is being able to abide with spiritual mystery while not knowing the answers. Maybe the answers can't come through your head but only through your heart. Maybe part of the mystery is that faith can renew itself over and over.

In the end, all I know for sure is gratitude.

And I thought about the last year—the odd flashes of pure joy, the constant fear that underlay my daily living and became acute with every freckle, cough, headache or misspoken word. And I thought, I am alive. Alive. Can anyone, anywhere, with any assurance, say more?
—Juliet Wittman, *Breast Cancer Journal,*
A Century of Petals

For some joy is not to be shared, not to be rendered down to a pool of expressed emotion. It bends over language, and the self bows down to it in serious awe . . . For now, the exile of the body is partly over, though the spiritual education by exile will not end . . . I take step after step into a new world, wild and joyous and fearful with possibility.
—Suzanne E. Berger, *Horizontal Woman*

A week ago I read again The Old Man and the Sea, *and learned from it that, above all, our bodies exist to perform the condition of our spirits: our choices, our desires, our loves. My physical mobility and my little girls have been taken from me; but I remain. So my crippling is a daily and living sculpture of certain truths: we receive and we lose, and we must try to achieve gratitude; and with that gratitude to embrace with whole hearts whatever of life that remains after the losses. No one can do this alone, for being absolutely alone finally means a life not only without people or God or both to love, but without love itself. In The Old Man and the Sea, Santiago is a widower and a man who prays; but the love that fills and sustains him is of life itself: living creatures, and the sky, and the sea. Without that love, he would be an old man alone on a boat.*

—Andre Dubus, *Broken Vessels*

Your own story—the small ordinary details of your life and the earth-shaking moments of upheaval and change, what you felt, where you went on this journey, what you saw, what you took with you, and what you left behind—is unique and precious. And you're the only one who can tell it.

Writing is a creative act relying on faith, and nothing can heal the spirit like creativity and faith. Faith that you have something to say and that you'll find the words to say it. Faith that there is meaning in each breath you take and in each small detail of your life and that this is worth writing about. Faith that others will find comfort and connection in your story.

Trust your deep well of memory and feeling, of observation and experience. Know that when you write the truth, it's simply the truth, your truth. There is no right or wrong way to record your life, to express your thoughts and your feelings. Just begin.

Relax. Don't think. Keep writing.

BIBLIOGRAPHY

Allende, Isabel. *Paula.* New York: HarperCollins, 1994

Armstrong, Lance (with Sally Jenkins). *It's Not About the Bike.* New York: G.P. Putnam's Sons, 2000

Bank, Melissa, *The Girls' Guide to Hunting and Fishing.* New York: Viking Penguin, 1999

Berger, Suzanne E. *Horizontal Woman.* Boston: Houghton Mifflin Company, 1996

Bolen, Jean Shinoda. *Close to the Bone, Life-Threatening Illness and the Search for Meaning.* New York: Scribner, 1996

Bradbury, Ray. *Zen In The Art of Writing, Essays on Creativity.* Santa Barbara, California: Capra Press, 1990

Brodie, Deborah (editor). *Writing Changes Everything.* New York: St. Martin's Press, 1997

Broyard, Anatole. *Intoxicated by My Illness.* New York: Clarkson Potter, 1992

Carver, Raymond. *A New Path to the Waterfall.* New York: The Atlantic Monthly Press, 1989

Coles, Robert. *The Call of Stories, Teaching and the Moral Imagination.* Boston: Houghton Mifflin Company, 1989

Collins, Nancy. "The Unsinkable Spirit of Michael J. Fox." *George,* October 2000

Conway, Kathlyn. *Ordinary Life, A Memoir of Illness.* New York: W. H. Freeman and Company, 1997

Cooper, Bernard. *Truth Serum.* New York: Houghton Mifflin Company, 1996

Couser, G. Thomas. *Recovering Bodies: Illness, Disability, and Life Writing.* Madison, Wisconsin: The University of Wisconsin Press, 1997

Cousins, Norman. *Anatomy of an Illness.* New York: W.W. Norton & Co., 1979

Dennis, Sandy. *A Personal Memoir.* Watsonville, California: Papier-Mache Press, 1997

De Salvo, Louise. *Writing As a Way of Healing.* San Francisco: HarperSanFrancisco, 1999

——*Breathless, An Asthma Journal.* Boston: Beacon Press, 1997

Dossey, Larry. *Healing Words.* San Francisco: HarperSanFrancisco, 1993

Doty, Mark. *Heaven's Coast, A Memoir.* New York: HarperCollins, 1996

Dubus, Andre. *Broken Vessels.* Boston: David R. Godine, 1991

Ehrlich, Gretel. *A Match to the Heart.* New York: Penguin Books, 1994

Eikenberry, Jill (introduction), Terry Tempest Williams (epilogue). *Art. Rage. Us.* San Francisco: Chronicle Books, 1998

Fisher, Mary. *My Name Is Mary.* New York: Scribner, 1996

Foster, Patricia and Swander, Mary. *The Healing Circle, Authors Writing of Recovery.* New York: Penguin Books, 1998

Frank, Arthur W. *The Wounded Storyteller, Body, Illness, and Ethics.* Chicago: The University of Chicago Press, 1997

Gilchrist, Ellen. *Falling Through Space.* Boston: Little, Brown & Company, 1987

Goldberg, Natalie. *Wild Mind, Living the Writer's Life.* New York: Bantam Books, 1990

Gurganus, Allan. *Plays Well with Others.* New York: Vintage Books, 1997

Hall, Donald. *Life Work.* Boston: Beacon Press, 1993

Haskell, Molly. *Love and Other Infectious Diseases.* New York: William Morrow and Company, 1990

Hockenberry, John. *Moving Violations.* New York: Hyperion, 1995

Hoffman, Alice. "Sustained by Fiction While Facing Life's Facts." *New York Times,* 8/14/00

King, Stephen. *On Writing, A Memoir of the Craft.* New York: Scribner, 2000

Korda, Michael. *Man to Man, Surviving Prostate Cancer.* New York: Random House, 1996

Kriegel, Leonard. *Flying Solo.* Boston: Beacon Press, 1998

Lamott, Anne. *Bird by Bird, Some Instructions on Writing and Life.* New York: Pantheon Books, 1994

Lee, Laurel. *Walking Through the Fire, A Hospital Journal.* New York: E. P. Dutton, 1977

Lipsett, Suzanne. *Surviving a Writer's Life.* San Francisco: HarperSanFrancisco, 1994

Lipsyte, Robert. *In The Country of Illness.* New York: Alfred K. Knopf, 1998

Lorde, Audre. *The Cancer Journals.* San Francisco: aunt lute books, 1980

Love, Susan M. *Dr. Susan Love's Breast Book.* New York: Addison-Wesley Publishing Company, 1996

Mairs, Nancy. *Plain Text.* Tucson, Arizona: The University of Arizona Press, 1986

Mayer, Musa. *Examining Myself: One Woman's Story of Breast Cancer Treatment and Recovery.* Boston: Faber and Faber, 1993

McCrum, Robert. *My Year Off, Recovering Life After A Stroke.* New York: W. W. Norton and Co., 1998

Metzger, Deena. *Writing for Your Life, A Guide and Companion to the Inner Worlds.* San Francisco: HarperSanFrancisco, 1992

Monette, Paul. *Borrowed Time, An AIDS Memoir.* New York: Harcourt Brace & Company, 1994

Morrow, Lance. "Lessons of a Bad Heart." *Time,* 3/19/01

Moyers, Bill. *Healing and the Mind.* New York: Doubleday, 1993

Myers, Art. *Winged Victory.* San Diego: Photographic Gallery of Fine Art Books, 1996

Nash, Jennie. *The Victoria's Secret Catalog Keeps Coming.* New York: Scribners, 2001

Nielsen, Jerri (with Maryanne Vollers). *Ice Bound, A Doctor's Incredible Battle for Survival at the South Pole.* New York: Hyperion, 2001

Oliver, Mary. *New and Selected Poems.* Boston: Beacon Press, 1992

Orenstein, Peggy. "Breast Cancer at 35." *New York Times Magazine,* 6/19/97

Parker, Joan H. and Robert B. *Three Weeks in Spring.* Boston: Houghton Mifflin Company, 1978

Pennebaker, James W. *Opening Up.* New York: Guilford Press, 1990

Pesmen, Curtis. "My Cancer Story." *Esquire,* September 2001

Price, Reynolds. *A Whole New Life.* New York: Atheneum, 1994

Radner, Gilda. *It's Always Something.* New York: Simon & Schuster, 1989

Raz, Hilda (editor). *Living on the Margins, Women Writers on Breast Cancer.* New York: Persea Books, 1999

Reeve, Christopher. *Still Me.* New York: The Ballantine Publishing Group, 1999

Rhett, Kathryn (editor). *Survival Stories, Memoirs of Crisis.* New York: Doubleday, 1997

Rosenbaum, Ernest H. and Isadora R., editors. *Inner Fire.* Austin, Texas: Plexus, 1999

Sarton, May. *After the Stroke.* New York: W. W. Norton & Company, 1988

Smyth, Joshua M., Arthur A. Stone, Adam Hurewitz, and Alan Kaell. "Effects of Writing About Stressful Experiences on Symptom Reduction in Patients with Asthma or Rheumatoid Arthritis." *Journal of the American Medical Association,* April 14, 1999

Sontag, Susan. *Illness as Metaphor.* New York: Farrar, Straus and Giroux, 1978

Sternburg, Janet, editor. *The Writer on Her Work.* New York: W. W. Norton & Company, 1980

Wadler, Joyce. *My Breast.* New York: Addison-Wesley Publishing Company, 1992

Winawer, Sidney, J., with Nick Taylor. *Healing Lessons.* New York: Little, Brown & Company, 1998

Wittman, Juliet. *Breast Cancer Journal, A Century of Petals.* Golden, Colorado: Fulcrum Publishing, 1993

ACKNOWLEDGMENTS

I want to acknowledge my deep debt to all the members of the writing workshop at The Wellness Community in Redondo Beach, California, and my gratitude for their courage, honesty, generosity, and infinite patience. To those members who gave me their writing exercises to include in this book, thank you for the gift of your words. Thanks also to those whose work does not appear in these pages because of their wish to keep it private, but whose presence in the workshop helped to influence and inspire the book.

Thanks to the three friends who have read and commented on all the many drafts of the manuscript: Norma Almquist, who started me on my writing path and shaped my reading taste, for her willingness to continue reading my pages thirty years after I took her creative writing courses. Debra Smith, for her humor and spirit, and generosity of time and good ideas. And especially Sally Court for telling me in the beginning to write it all down, and for her wisdom in knowing what was needed and what was not.

Thanks to friends who read the early pages and offered encouraging comments: Billy Mernit, Jeanne Nichols, Laura Fisher Smith, Phyllis Glick-Berger, Sue Kane, and especially my husband. And to Paula Diamond for her take-no-prisoners e-mail messages.

Thanks to Linda Venis, director of The Writers' Program at UCLA Extension, for her support and eloquent notes, and also for creating an atmosphere that makes teaching creative writing at UCLA Extension one of the great pleasures and learning experiences of life.

Thanks to Judith Opdahl and her staff at The Wellness Community, especially Ruth Crandell, inspiration to us all, and to Linda Neal for allowing me to include her writing.

Thanks to the Bosom Buddies. Their names have been changed in this book, but they know who they are and how important they have been to me, and continue to be.

Thanks to Aaron Priest for years of good advice and for saying yes to this book, to Lisa Erbach Vance who found the perfect editor and publisher for it, for her dedication and tenacity, and to Alicia Brooks, my editor, for her belief in the book from the very beginning, for her enthusiasm and constant encouragement, and for making the editing of it so much fun. Thanks also to my publisher at Griffin, Matthew Shear, and to Griffin product manager Karen Tepper and production editor extraordinaire Kevin Sweeney.

To my daughters, Brooke and Gillan, and my granddaughter, Emma—thank you for bringing so much joy and light into my life. I love you.

In memory—Patti Tate and Margie Lemen
    . . . and each body a lion of courage, and something precious to the earth.
                              —Mary Oliver from "When Death Comes"

A portion of the profits of this book is donated to The Wellness Community—South Bay Cities in Redondo Beach, California.

ABOUT THE AUTHOR

BARBARA ABERCROMBIE lives in Santa Monica, California, with her husband. She has published two novels, books for children, and numerous poems, articles, and personal essays. She teaches in The Writers' Program at UCLA Extension, where she won the 1994 Outstanding Teacher Award. She also conducts ongoing writing workshops at The Wellness Community, a nationwide program that offers free psychological support for cancer patients and their families.

PERMISSIONS

The author and publisher wish to thank the following publishers, authors, agents, and publications:

Beacon Press, Boston, for permission to use a quote from *Flying Solo* by Leonard Kriegel, copyright © 1998 by Leonard Kriegel, to quote from *Life Work* by Donald Hall, copyright © 1993 by Donald Hall, and to use excerpts from *New and Selected Poems* by Mary Oliver, copyright © 1992 Mary Oliver.

BOA Editions, Ltd., for permission to reprint "1994" by Lucille Clifton from *Blessing the Boats, New and Selected Poems,* copyright © 2000, 1996 by Lucille Clifton.

Georges Borchardt, Inc., agent for the author, for permission to use an excerpt from *Love and Other Infectious Diseases* by Molly Haskell, copyright © 1990 by Molly Haskell.

Clarkson Potter Publishers, a division of Random House, Inc., for permission to use excerpts from *Intoxicated by My Illness* by Anatole Broyard, copyright © 1992 by the Estate of Anatole Broyard.

Kathlyn Conway for permission to use excerpts from her book *Ordinary Life, A Memoir of Illness,* published by W. H. Freeman and Company, copyright © 1997 by W. H. Freeman and Company, copyright © 2002 Kathlyn Conway.

Doubleday, a division of Random House, Inc., for permission to quote from *Healing and the Mind* by Bill Moyers, copyright © 1993 by Public Affairs Television, Inc., and David Grubin Productions, Inc.

David R. Godine, Publisher, Inc., for permission to quote from *Broken Vessels* by Andre Dubus, copyright © 1991 by Andre Dubus.

The Estate of Sandra Dale Dennis for permission to use excerpts from *Sandy Dennis, A Personal Memoir* by Sandy Dennis, co-edited by Louise Ladd and Doug Taylor,